EDITION

3

CLINICAL CALCULATIONS MADE EASY

Solving Problems Using Dimensional Analysis

Gloria P. Craig, RN, MSN, EdD
Department Head, Nursing Student Services
Coordinator, Continuing Nursing Education
Associate Professor
South Dakota State University
College of Nursing
Brookings, South Dakota

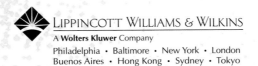
LIPPINCOTT WILLIAMS & WILKINS
A **Wolters Kluwer** Company
Philadelphia • Baltimore • New York • London
Buenos Aires • Hong Kong • Sydney • Tokyo

Senior Acquisitions Editor: Margaret Zuccarini
Managing Editor: Helen Kogut
Editorial Assistant: Carol DeVault
Production Editor: Danielle Michaely
Director of Nursing Production: Helen Ewan
Managing Editor/Production: Erika Kors
Art Director: Carolyn O'Brien
Senior Manufacturing Manager: William Alberti
Indexer: Victoria Boyle
Compositor: Circle Graphics
Printer: R.R. Donnelley—Willard

Third Edition

Library of Congress Cataloging-in-Publication Data

Craig, Gloria P., 1949-
  Clinical calculations made easy : solving problems using dimensional analysis / Gloria P. Craig.—Ed. 3.
     p. ; cm.
  Includes bibliographical references and index.
  ISBN 0-7817-4838-0 (alk. paper)
  1. Pharmaceutical arithmetic. 2. Dimensional analysis. 3. Nursing—Mathematics. I. Title.
  [DNLM: 1. Pharmaceutical Preparations—administration & dosage—Nurses' Instruction. 2. Pharmaceutical Preparations—administration & dosage—Problems and Exercises. 3. Mathematics—Nurses' Instruction. 4. Mathematics—Problems and Exercises. 5. Problem Solving—Nurses' Instruction. 6. Problem Solving—Problems and Exercises. QV 748 C886ca 2005]
  RS57.C73 2005
  615'.14—dc22

                                                                          2004044146

Care has been taken to confirm the accuracy of the information presented and to describe generally accepted practices. However, the authors, editors, and publisher are not responsible for errors or omissions or for any consequences from application of the information in this book and make no warranty, express or implied, with respect to the content of the publication.

The authors, editors, and publisher have exerted every effort to ensure that drug selection and dosage set forth in this text are in accordance with the current recommendations and practice at the time of publication. However, in view of ongoing research, changes in government regulations, and the constant flow of information relating to drug therapy and drug reactions, the reader is urged to check the package insert for each drug for any change in indications and dosage and for added warnings and precautions. This is particularly important when the recommended agent is a new or infrequently employed drug.

Some drugs and medical devices presented in this publication have Food and Drug Administration (FDA) clearance for limited use in restricted research settings. It is the responsibility of the health care provider to ascertain the FDA status of each drug or device planned for use in his or her clinical practice.

LWW.com

Reviewers

Jamie L. Flower, MS, SANE, RN
Assistant Professor
University of Arkansas at Fort Smith
Fort Smith, Arkansas

Stephanie J. Guy, BSN, RN
LPN Instructor
Southeast Arkansas College
Pine Bluff, Arkansas

Regina Janoski, BC, MSN, RN
Assistant Professor of Nursing
Montgomery County Community College
Blue Bell, Pennsylvania

Janice M. Jones, PhD, RN, CNS
Clinical Assistant Professor of Nursing
University of Buffalo, School of Nursing
Buffalo, New York

Ruth Klawiter, MS, RN
Instructor
South Dakota State University
Brookings, South Dakota

Lauren O'Hare, EdD, RN
Assistant Professor of Nursing
Wagner College
Staten Island, New York

Peggy Przybycien, MS, RN
Associate Professor
Onondaga Community College
Syracuse, New York

Preface

Many people experience stumbling blocks calculating math problems because of a lack of mathematical ability or associated "math anxiety." Even people with strong math skills often set up medication problems incorrectly, putting the patient at an increased risk for incorrect dosages and the ensuing consequences. However, dosage calculation need not be difficult if you use a problem-solving method that is easy to understand and to implement.

As a student, I experienced anxiety related to poor mathematical abilities and consequently had difficulty with medication calculations. However, a friend introduced me to a problem-solving method that was easy to visualize. By using this method, I was able to easily understand medication problems and thereby avoid the stumbling blocks that I had experienced with other methods of dosage calculations. Later, as a practicing nurse and nursing instructor, I realized that many of my colleagues and students shared my experience with "math anxiety," so I began sharing this problem-solving method with them.

During my baccalaureate nursing education, this problem-solving method became my teaching plan. During my master's education, it became my research. During my doctoral education, it became my dissertation. Now, I would like to share this method with anyone who ever believed that they were mathematically "challenged" or trembled at the thought of solving a medication problem.

The method, called dimensional analysis (also known as factor-label method or conversion-factor method), is a systematic, straightforward approach to setting up and solving problems that require conversions. It is a way of thinking about problems that can be used when two quantities are directly proportional to each other, but one needs to be converted using a conversion factor in order for the problem to be solved.

Dimensional Analysis as a Teaching Tool

Dimensional analysis empowers the learner to solve a variety of medication problems using just one problem-solving method. Research has shown that students experience less frustration and create fewer **medication errors** if one problem-solving method is used to solve **all** medication problems. As a method of reducing errors and improving calculation **abilities,** dimensional analysis has many possibilities. Whether it is used in practice or education, it is a strong approach when the goals are improving medication dosage-calculation skills, reducing medication errors, and improving patient safety. Ultimately, this improved methodology has the potential to reduce the medication errors that occur within the discipline of nursing.

Dimensional analysis helps the learner see and understand the significance of the whole process, since it focuses on how to learn, rather than what to learn. It provides a framework for understanding the principles of the problem-solving method and supports the critical thinking process. It helps the learner to organize and evaluate data, and to avoid errors in setting up problems. Dimensional analysis thus supports the conceptual mastery and higher-level

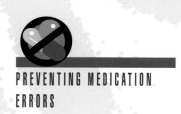

PREVENTING MEDICATION ERRORS

thinking skills that have become the core of curricula at all levels of nursing education.

Organization of This Book

The book is divided into four sections: Section 1 provides instruction and explanation for students learning to solve clinical calculations problems by using dimensional analysis, Section 2 provides practice problems for students to strengthen their skills; Section 3 contains 25 case studies to help students relate their skills to clinical situations, and Section 4 contains a comprehensive Post-Test.

Section 1: Clinical Calculations

This text uses the simple-to-complex approach to teach students clinical calculations. The first chapter provides a review of basic arithmetic skills, while the second chapter reviews systems of measurement and common equivalents. The third chapter introduces students to dimensional analysis and allows them to build upon Chapter 2 by using common equivalents to practice their dimensional analysis skills. Finally, Chapters 4 to 6 teach clinical calculations, starting with One-Factor Conversions (Chapter 4), then Two-Factor Conversions (Chapter 5), and finally Three-Factor Conversions (Chapter 6).

Similarly, each chapter uses the simple-to-complex approach to the material. As the learner continues through the text, more complex concepts are presented. Each chapter contains numerous examples with detailed explanations, including a special **Thinking It Through** feature, to enhance student learning. **In-chapter exercises,** which occur after the presentation and explanation of each new concept, provide an opportunity for the learner to gain ability and build confidence in the material before proceeding to the next concept. To provide the learner with the clinically realistic examples, **actual drug labels** are liberally used as the basis of medication problems. Near the end of each chapter are **practice problems,** where the students can practice their skills and assess mastery of the material to identify any areas where more review is necessary.

The answers to all of the exercises and the practice problems are located at the end of each chapter in an **answer key,** for easy reference for students. The answer section also provides a complete explanation for each problem by showing exactly how the problem was set up and then solved.

Finally, each chapter concludes with a **post-test,** a resource for instructors to evaluate their students' understanding of the concepts presented in that chapter. The post-tests are designed so that the students may work on them, tear them out of the book, and hand them in. The answers to the post-tests are in the Instructor's Manual.

Section 2: Practice Problems

This section allows students to refine their skills in each area. The three parts are one-, two-, and three-factor practice problems, respectively, and a final section on comprehensive questions. An answer key at the end of this section contains answers and explanations for all of the problems.

Section 3: Case Studies

This section contains 25 case studies, related to different fields of nursing. The purpose of the case studies is to help students relate their clinical calculation skills to clinical situations.

Section 4: Comprehensive Post-Test

The last section of the book contains a post-test of 20 questions allowing the instructor to assess students' mastery of solving clinical calculations using dimensional analysis. The answers to these questions are found in the Instructor's Manual.

Third Edition

The third edition of ***Clinical Calculations Made Easy: Solving Problems Using Dimensional Analysis*** continues to enhance the visual appeal of the book, making it more "user-friendly." The second edition was designed in four colors to make the text more visually interesting and to allow reprinting of actual drug labels to more closely simulate the real clinical experience of the nurse. The size of the book was enlarged to a workbook size to provide more opportunities for students to practice their medication calculation skills.

The third edition revision introduces three important new features:

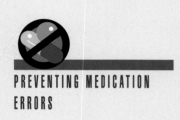

PREVENTING MEDICATION ERRORS

Medication Error Prevention

The third edition highlights methods that assist in **preventing medication errors** that continue to plague the health profession. An icon is included throughout the text to identify key concepts necessary for the prevention of medication errors. Each chapter highlights methods of medication error prevention as it applies to the content in that chapter.

Pediatric Medication Problems

A second new feature for the third edition is the inclusion of an icon to identify **pediatric medication problems.** Many teachers like to have the opportunity to focus on content for a particular area. Although the majority of the medication problems in the text are calculated for an adult, teachers and students will now be able to quickly identify all pediatric problems by searching for the pediatric feature icon.

More Dosage Calculation Problems

The third edition provides more opportunities for students to practice their skills. More **dosage calculation problems** have been added to selected chapters and to the **CD-ROM** in the back of the book.

Finally, **five new case studies** have been added to the text. The 25 case studies include medication problems from all clinical areas including medical-surgical, pediatric, obstetrics, and mental health.

It is my hope that this new edition will help nursing students and other health care professionals find that clinical calculation can indeed be made easy using dimensional analysis.

Gloria P. Craig

Acknowledgments

There are many people who have assisted me with my professional growth and development, including:

- **Pauline Callahan,** who believed that I would be a great nurse and nursing instructor when I could not believe in myself.

- **Jackie Kehm,** who introduced me to dimensional analysis and helped me pass the medication module that I was sure would be my stumbling block.

- **Dr. Sandra L. Sellers,** for her expertise and guidance throughout the process of writing my thesis and her encouragement to write a textbook.

- **Margaret Cooper,** for her friendship and editing support throughout the writing of this textbook.

- My students, colleagues, and reviewers, for helping me develop my abilities to explain and teach the problem-solving method of dimensional analysis.

- The numerous pharmaceutical companies listed throughout this book that supplied medication labels and gave permission for the labels to be included in this textbook.

- The faculty at South Dakota State University, College of Nursing, for allowing dimensional analysis to be integrated into the curriculum as the problem-solving method for medication calculation.

- The Lippincott editorial and production teams, for all of their hard work: **Margaret Zuccarini,** Senior Acquisitions Editor; **Helen Kogut,** Managing Editor; **Danielle Michaely,** Production Editor; and **Carolyn O'Brien,** Art Director.

To these people and many more, I would like to express my sincere appreciation for their mentoring, guidance, support, and encouragement that have helped to turn a dream into a reality.

This third edition of my text is dedicated to my children, **Lori and Randy,** and to my granddaughters, **Zoë and Ava.**

Contents

SECTION 1
Clinical Calculations   1

CHAPTER 1   **Arithmetic Review   3**

Arabic Numbers and Roman Numerals   4
    Exercise 1.1   Arabic Numbers and Roman Numerals   5

Fractions   7
Multiplying Fractions   8
    Exercise 1.2   Multiplying Fractions   8
Dividing Fractions   9
    Exercise 1.3   Dividing Fractions   10

Decimals   11
Rounding Decimals   11
    Exercise 1.4   Rounding Decimals   12
Multiplying Decimals   12
    Exercise 1.5   Multiplying Decimals   12
Dividing Decimals   13
    Exercise 1.6   Dividing Decimals   14
Converting Fractions to Decimals   14
    Exercise 1.7   Converting Fractions to Decimals   15
Practice Problems   16
Post-Test   19
Answer Key   21

CHAPTER 2   **Systems of Measurement and Common Equivalents   29**

Systems of Measurement   30
The Metric System   30
The Apothecary System   31
The Household System   32
Temperature   33
Common Equivalents   34
Practice Problems   34
Post-Test   37
Answer Key   39

CHAPTER 3   **Solving Problems Using Dimensional Analysis   41**

Terms Used in Dimensional Analysis   42

The Five Steps of Dimensional Analysis   42
    Exercise 3.1   Dimensional Analysis   46
Practice Problems   49
Post-Test   51
Answer Key   53

CHAPTER 4   **One-Factor Medication Problems   59**

Interpretation of Medication Orders   60
Right Patient   60
Right Drug   60
Right Dosage   60
Right Route   61
Right Time   61
    Exercise 4.1   Interpretation of Medication Orders   61
One-Factor Medication Problems   62
Principles of Rounding   65
    Exercise 4.2   One-Factor Medication Problems   68
Components of a Drug Label   68
Identifying the Components   68
    Exercise 4.3   Identifying the Components of Drug Labels   69
Solving Problems With Components of Drug Labels   71
    Exercise 4.4   Problems With Components of Drug Labels   73
Administering Medication by Different Routes   74
Enteral Medications   74
    Exercise 4.5   Administering Enteral Medications   79
Parenteral Medications   80
    Exercise 4.6   Administering Parenteral Medications   85
Practice Problems   87
Post-Test   91
Answer Key   97

CHAPTER 5   **Two-Factor Medication Problems   103**

Medication Problems Involving Weight   104
    Exercise 5.1   Pediatric Medication Problems Involving Weight   106

Medication Problems Involving Reconstitution 108

> Exercise 5.2   Medication Problems Involving Reconstitution   111

Medication Problems Involving Intravenous Pumps 112

> Exercise 5.3   Medication Problems Involving Intravenous Pumps   115

Medication Problems Involving Drop Factors 116

> Exercise 5.4   Medication Problems Involving Drop Factors   120

Medication Problems Involving Intermittent Infusion 120

> Exercise 5.5   Medication Problems Involving Intermittent Infusion   122

Practice Problems 124
Post-Test 127
Answer Key 131

CHAPTER 6   **Three-Factor Medication Problems 137**

> Exercise 6.1   Medication Problems Involving Dosage, Weight, and Time   144

Practice Problems 150
Post-Test 153
Answer Key 159

SECTION 2
Practice Problems 163

One-Factor Practice Problems 165
Two-Factor Practice Problems 179
Three-Factor Practice Problems 190
Comprehensive Practice Problems 195
Answer Key 199

SECTION 3
Case Studies 211

CASE STUDY 1:   **Congestive Heart Failure 213**
CASE STUDY 2:   **COPD/Emphysema 214**
CASE STUDY 3:   **Small Cell Lung Cancer 215**

CASE STUDY 4:   **Acquired Immunodeficiency Syndrome (AIDS) 216**
CASE STUDY 5:   **Sickle Cell Anemia 217**
CASE STUDY 6:   **Deep Vein Thrombosis 217**
CASE STUDY 7:   **Bone Marrow Transplant 218**
CASE STUDY 8:   **Pneumonia 219**
CASE STUDY 9:   **Pain 220**
CASE STUDY 10:   **Cirrhosis 221**
CASE STUDY 11:   **Hyperemesis Gravidarum 221**
CASE STUDY 12:   **Preeclampsia 222**
CASE STUDY 13:   **Premature Labor 223**
CASE STUDY 14:   **Cystic Fibrosis 224**
CASE STUDY 15:   **Respiratory Syncytial Virus (RSV) 225**
CASE STUDY 16:   **Leukemia 226**
CASE STUDY 17:   **Sepsis 227**
CASE STUDY 18:   **Bronchopulmonary Dysplasia 228**
CASE STUDY 19:   **Cerebral Palsy 229**
CASE STUDY 20:   **Hyperbilirubinemia 230**
CASE STUDY 21:   **Spontaneous Abortion 231**
CASE STUDY 22:   **Bipolar Disorder 232**
CASE STUDY 23:   **Anorexia Nervosa 232**
CASE STUDY 24:   **Clinical Depression 233**
CASE STUDY 25:   **Alzheimer's Disease 234**
Answer Key 235

SECTION 4
Comprehensive Post-Test 245

APPENDIX
Educational Theory of Dimensional Analysis 251

Index 255

1

Clinical
Calculations

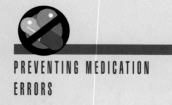

PREVENTING MEDICATION ERRORS

Every nurse must know and practice the five rights of medication administration including the

1. Right drug
2. Right dose
3. Right route
4. Right time
5. Right patient

Although the right drug, route, time, and patient may be readily identified, the right dose requires **arithmetic skills** that may be difficult for you. This chapter reviews the basic arithmetic skills (multiplication and division) **necessary for calculating** medication dosage problems using the problem-solving method of dimensional analysis. Calculating the **right dose** of medication to be administered to a patient is one of the first steps toward preventing **medication errors.**

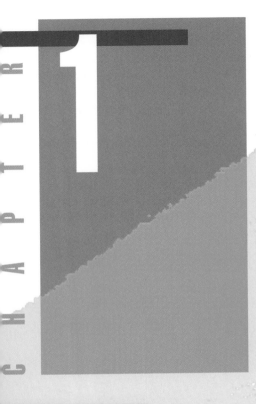

Arithmetic Review

Outline

**ARABIC NUMBERS
AND ROMAN NUMERALS 4**
Exercise 1.1: Arabic Numbers
and Roman Numerals 5
FRACTIONS 7
Multiplying Fractions 8
Exercise 1.2: Multiplying Fractions 8
Dividing Fractions 9
Exercise 1.3: Dividing Fractions 10
DECIMALS 11
Rounding Decimals 11
Exercise 1.4: Rounding Decimals 12
Multiplying Decimals 12
Exercise 1.5: Multiplying Decimals 12
Dividing Decimals 13
Exercise 1.6: Dividing Decimals 14
**CONVERTING FRACTIONS
TO DECIMALS 14**
Exercise 1.7: Converting Fractions
to Decimals 15
**Practice Problems for Chapter 1:
Arithmetic Review 16**
**Post-Test for Chapter 1:
Arithmetic Review 19**
**Answer Key for Chapter 1:
Arithmetic Review 21**

Objectives

After completing this chapter, you will be able to:

1. Express Arabic numbers as Roman numerals.
2. Express Roman numerals as Arabic numbers.
3. Identify the numerator and denominator in a fraction.
4. Multiply and divide fractions.
5. Multiply and divide decimals.
6. Convert fractions to decimals.

■ ARABIC NUMBERS AND ROMAN NUMERALS

Most medication dosages are ordered by the physician or the nurse practitioner in the metric and household systems for weights and measures using the Arabic number system with symbols called **digits** (ie, 1, 2, 3, 4, 5). Occasionally, orders are received in the apothecary system of weights and measures using the Roman numeral system with numbers represented by **symbols** (ie, I, V, X). The Roman numeral system uses seven basic symbols, and various combinations of these symbols represent all numbers in the Arabic number system.

Table 1.1 includes the seven basic Roman numerals and the corresponding Arabic numbers.

The combination of Roman numeral symbols is based on three specific principles:

1. Symbols are used to construct a number, but no symbol may be used more than three times. The exception is the symbol for five (V), which is used only once because there is a symbol for 10 (X) and a combination of symbols for 15 (XV).

EXAMPLE 1.1

$$III = (1 + 1 + 1) = 3$$
$$XXX = (10 + 10 + 10) = 30$$

2. When symbols of lesser value follow symbols of greater value, they are *added* to construct a number.

EXAMPLE 1.2

$$VIII = (5 + 3) = 8$$
$$XVII = (10 + 5 + 1 + 1) = 17$$

■ TABLE 1.1 Seven Basic Roman Numerals	
ROMAN NUMERALS	**ARABIC NUMBERS**
I	1
V	5
X	10
L	50
C	100
D	500
M	1000

3. When symbols of greater value follow symbols of lesser value, those of lesser value are *subtracted* from those of higher value to construct a number.

EXAMPLE 1.3

IV = (5 - 1) = 4
IX = (10 - 1) = 9

Exercise 1.1 **Arabic Numbers and Roman Numerals**
(See page 21 for answers)

Express the following Arabic numbers as Roman numerals.

1. 1 = I
2. 2 = II
3. 3 = III
4. 4 = IV
5. 5 = V
6. 6 = VI
7. 7 = VII
8. 8 = VIII
9. 9 = VIIII
10. 10 = X
11. 11 = XI
12. 12 = XII
13. 13 = XIII
14. 14 = XIIII
15. 15 = XV
16. 16 = XVI
17. 17 = XVII
18. 18 = XVIII
19. 19 = _____
20. 20 = _____

(Exercise continues on page 6)

Although medication orders rarely involve Roman numerals higher than 20, for additional practice, express the following Arabic numbers as Roman numerals.

21. 43 = _____

22. 24 = _____

23. 55 = _____

24. 32 = _____

25. 102 = _____

26. 150 = _____

27. 75 = _____

28. 92 = _____

29. 64 = _____

30. 69 = _____

Express the following Roman numerals as Arabic numbers.

31. II   = _____

32. IV   = _____

33. VI   = _____

34. X   = _____

35. VIII = _____

36. XIX   = _____

37. XX   = _____

38. XVIII = _____

39. I   = _____

40. XV   = _____

41. III   = _____

42. V   = _____

43. IX   = _____

44. VII   = _____

45. XI   = _____

46. XIV   = _____

47. XVI   = _____

48. XII   = _____

49. XVII = _____

50. XIII = _____

To increase your abilities to use either system, convert the following Arabic numbers or Roman numerals.

51. 19 = _____

52. XII = _____

53. 7 = _____

54. IX = _____

55. IV = _____

56. 11 = _____

57. VIII = _____

58. 16 = _____

59. XX = _____

60. 5 = _____

61. I = _____

62. 18 = _____

63. VI = _____

64. 2 = _____

65. III = _____

66. 10 = _____

67. XIII = _____

68. 14 = _____

69. XV = _____

70. 17 = _____

■ FRACTIONS

Medication dosages with fractions are occasionally ordered by the physician or used by the pharmaceutical manufacturer on the drug label. A **fraction** is a number that represents part of a whole number and contains three parts:

1. **Numerator**—the number on the top portion of the fraction that represents the number of parts of the whole fraction.
2. **Dividing line**—the line separating the top portion of the fraction from the bottom portion of the fraction.
3. **Denominator**—the number on the bottom portion of the fraction that represents the number of parts into which the whole is divided.

$$\frac{3}{4} = \frac{\text{numerator}}{\text{denominator}}$$

PREVENTING MEDICATION ERRORS

Understanding fractions will assist in preventing **medication errors.** A medication order may include a fraction.

Example: Administer 1/150 gr of nitroglycerin.

To solve medication dosage calculation problems using dimensional analysis, you must be able to identify the numerator and denominator portion of the problem. You also must be able to multiply and divide numbers, fractions, and decimals.

Multiplying Fractions

The three steps for multiplying fractions are:

1. Multiply the numerators.
2. Multiply the denominators.
3. Reduce the product to the lowest possible fraction.

EXAMPLE 1.4

$$\frac{2}{4} \times \frac{1}{8} = \frac{2}{32} = \frac{1}{16}$$

or

$$\frac{2 \text{ (numerator)}}{4 \text{ (denominator)}} \times \frac{1 \text{ (numerator)}}{8 \text{ (denominator)}} = \frac{2 \text{ (numerator)}}{32 \text{ (denominator)}}$$

$$= \frac{1}{16} \text{ (reduced to lowest possible fraction)}$$

EXAMPLE 1.5

$$\frac{1}{2} \times \frac{2}{4} = \frac{2}{8} = \frac{1}{4}$$

or

$$\frac{1 \text{ (numerator)}}{2 \text{ (denominator)}} \times \frac{2 \text{ (numerator)}}{4 \text{ (denominator)}} = \frac{2 \text{ (numerator)}}{8 \text{ (denominator)}}$$

$$= \frac{1}{4} \text{ (reduced to lowest possible fraction)}$$

Exercise 1.2   **Multiplying Fractions**
(See pages 21–22 for answers)

To increase your abilities when working with fractions, multiply the following fractions and reduce to the lowest fractional term.

1. $\dfrac{3}{4} \times \dfrac{5}{8} =$ $\dfrac{15}{40}$ $\dfrac{3}{8}$

2. $\dfrac{1}{3} \times \dfrac{4}{9} =$ $\dfrac{4}{27}$

3. $\dfrac{2}{3} \times \dfrac{4}{5} = \dfrac{8}{15}$

4. $\dfrac{3}{4} \times \dfrac{1}{2} =$

5. $\dfrac{1}{8} \times \dfrac{4}{5} =$

6. $\dfrac{2}{3} \times \dfrac{5}{8} =$

7. $\dfrac{3}{8} \times \dfrac{2}{3} =$

8. $\dfrac{4}{7} \times \dfrac{2}{4} =$

9. $\dfrac{4}{5} \times \dfrac{1}{2} =$

10. $\dfrac{1}{4} \times \dfrac{1}{8} =$

Dividing Fractions

The four steps for dividing fractions are:

1. Invert (turn upside down) the divisor portion of the problem (the second fraction in the problem).
2. Multiply the two numerators.
3. Multiply the two denominators.
4. Reduce answer to lowest term (fraction or whole number).

EXAMPLE 1.6

$$\frac{2}{4} \div \frac{1}{8} = \frac{2}{4} \times \frac{8}{1} = \frac{16}{4} = 4$$

or

$$\frac{2 \text{ (numerator)}}{4 \text{ (denominator)}} \div \frac{1 \text{ (numerator)}}{8 \text{ (denominator)}}$$

$$= \frac{2 \text{ (numerator)} \quad \times \quad 8 \text{ (numerator)}}{4 \text{ (denominator)} \times 1 \text{ (denominator)}} \begin{array}{c} \text{(inverted fraction)} \\ = 16 \\ = 4 \end{array}$$

$= 4$ (answer reduced to lowest term)

EXAMPLE 1.7

$$\frac{1}{2} \div \frac{2}{4} = \frac{1}{2} \times \frac{4}{2} = \frac{4}{4} = 1$$

or

$$\frac{1 \text{ (numerator)}}{2 \text{ (denominator)}} \div \frac{2 \text{ (numerator)}}{4 \text{ (denominator)}}$$

$$\qquad\qquad\qquad\quad \text{(inverted fraction)}$$

$$= \frac{1 \text{ (numerator)} \times 4 \text{ (numerator)}}{2 \text{ (denominator)} \times 2 \text{ (denominator)}} = \frac{4}{4}$$

$$= 1 \text{ (answer reduced to lowest term)}$$

Exercise 1.3   **Dividing Fractions**
(See page 22 for answers)

To increase your abilities when working with fractions, divide the following fractions and reduce to the lowest fractional term.

1. $\dfrac{3}{4} \div \dfrac{2}{3} =$

2. $\dfrac{1}{9} \div \dfrac{3}{9} =$

3. $\dfrac{2}{3} \div \dfrac{1}{6} =$

4. $\dfrac{1}{5} \div \dfrac{4}{5} =$

5. $\dfrac{3}{6} \div \dfrac{4}{8} =$

6. $\dfrac{5}{8} \div \dfrac{5}{8} =$

7. $\dfrac{1}{8} \div \dfrac{2}{3} =$

8. $\dfrac{1}{5} \div \dfrac{1}{2} =$

9. $\dfrac{1}{4} \div \dfrac{1}{2} =$

10. $\dfrac{1}{6} \div \dfrac{1}{3} =$

■ DECIMALS

Medication orders are often written using decimals, and pharmaceutical manufacturers may use decimals when labeling medications. Therefore, you must understand the learning principles involving decimals and be able to multiply and divide decimals.

- A decimal point is preceded by a zero if not preceded by a number to decrease the chance of an error if the decimal point is missed.

EXAMPLE 1.8

0.25

- A decimal point may be preceded by a number and followed by a number.

EXAMPLE 1.9

1.25

- Numbers to the left of the decimal point are *units, tens, hundreds, thousands,* and *ten-thousands.*
- Numbers to the right of the decimal point are *tenths, hundredths, thousandths,* and *ten-thousandths.*

EXAMPLE 1.10

```
    0.2 = 2 tenths
   0.05 = 5 hundredths
   0.25 = 25 hundredths
   1.25 = 1 unit and 25 hundredths
 110.25 = 110 units and 25 hundredths
```

Rounding Decimals

- Decimals may be rounded off. If the number to the right of the decimal is greater than or equal to 5 (≥ 5), round up to the next number.
- If the number to the right of the decimal is less than 5 (<5), delete the remaining numbers.

PREVENTING MEDICATION ERRORS

Understanding the importance of a decimal point will assist in preventing **medication errors.** An improper placement of a decimal point can result in a serious medication error.

Example: Administer 0.125 mg of Lanoxin.

If the "zero" is not placed in front of the decimal point the order could be misread.

Example: Administer 125 mg of Lanoxin.

EXAMPLE 1.11

0.78 → 0.8
0.213 → 0.2

Exercise 1.4   **Rounding Decimals**
(See page 22 for answers)

Practice rounding off the following decimals to the tenth.

1. 0.75 =

2. 0.88 =

3. 0.44 =

4. 0.23 =

5. 0.67 =

6. 0.27 =

7. 0.98 =

8. 0.92 =

9. 0.64 =

10. 0.250 =

Multiplying Decimals

When multiplying with decimals, the principles of multiplication still apply. The numbers are multiplied in columns, but the number of decimal points are counted and placed in the answer, counting places from right to left.

THINKING IT THROUGH

The answer to the problem before adding decimal points is 345 but when decimal points are correctly added (two decimal points are added to the answer, counting two places from the right to the left) then 3.45 becomes the correct answer.

EXAMPLE 1.12

$$\begin{array}{r} 2.3 \ (1\ \text{decimal point}) \\ \times 1.5 \ (1\ \text{decimal point}) \\ \hline 115 \\ 230 \\ \hline 3.45 \end{array}$$

Exercise 1.5   **Multiplying Decimals**
(See pages 22–23 for answers)

Practice multiplying the following decimals.

1.   2.5
    ×4.6

2.   1.45
   × 0.25

3.   3.9
   × 0.8

4.   2.56
   × 0.45

5.   10.65
   ×   0.05

6.   1.98
   × 3.10

7.   2.75
   × 5.0

8.   5.0
   × 0.45

9.   7.50
   × 0.25

10.   2.5
   × 0.01

Dividing Decimals

When dividing with decimals, the principles of division still apply, except that the dividing number is changed to a whole number by moving the decimal point to the right. The number being divided also changes by accepting the same number of decimal point moves.

EXAMPLE 1.13

$$0.5\overline{)0.75}$$

▶ **STEP 1 Move decimal point one place to the right.**

▶ **STEP 2**

$$
\begin{array}{r}
1.5 \\
5\overline{)7.5} \\
\underline{5} \\
2\,5 \\
\underline{2\,5} \\
0
\end{array}
$$

▶▶▶ *1.5*

Exercise 1.6   **Dividing Decimals**
(See pages 23–24 for answers)

Practice dividing the following decimals and rounding the answers to the tenth.

1. $3.4\overline{)9.6}$

2. $0.25\overline{)12.50}$

3. $0.56\overline{)18.65}$

4. $0.3\overline{)0.192}$

5. $0.4\overline{)12.43}$

6. $0.5\overline{)12.50}$

7. $0.125\overline{)0.25}$

8. $0.08\overline{)0.085}$

9. $1.5\overline{)22.5}$

10. $5.5\overline{)16.5}$

■ CONVERTING FRACTIONS TO DECIMALS

When problem solving with dimensional analysis, medication dosage calculation problems may frequently contain both fractions and decimals. Some of you may have fraction phobia and prefer to convert fractions to decimals when solving problems. To convert a fraction to a decimal, divide the numerator portion of the fraction by the denominator portion of the fraction.

When dividing fractions, remember to add a decimal point and a zero if the numerator cannot be divided by the denominator.

PREVENTING MEDICATION ERRORS

Understanding the importance of converting fractions to decimals will assist in preventing **medication errors.** Many medication errors occur because of a simple arithmetic error with dividing. Every nurse should have a calculator to recheck answers for accuracy.

EXAMPLE 1.14

$$\frac{1}{2} \text{ or } \frac{1 \text{ (numerator)}}{2 \text{ (denominator)}} = 2\overline{\smash{)}1.0} \quad \begin{array}{c} 0.5 = 0.5 \\ \underline{1\ 0} \end{array}$$

EXAMPLE 1.15

$$\frac{3}{4} \text{ or } \frac{3 \text{ (numerator)}}{4 \text{ (denominator)}} = 4\overline{\smash{\big)}3.00} \begin{array}{r} 0.75 \\ \hline 3.00 \\ \underline{2\ 8} \\ 20 \\ \underline{20} \end{array} = 0.75$$

Exercise 1.7   **Converting Fractions to Decimals**
(See pages 24–25 for answers)

To decrease fraction phobia, practice converting the following fractions to decimals. Remember to follow the rules of rounding.

1. $\dfrac{1}{8}$ =

2. $\dfrac{1}{4}$ =

3. $\dfrac{2}{5}$ =

4. $\dfrac{3}{5}$ =

5. $\dfrac{2}{3}$ =

6. $\dfrac{6}{8}$ =

7. $\dfrac{3}{8}$ =

8. $\dfrac{1}{3}$ =

9. $\dfrac{3}{6}$ =

10. $\dfrac{2}{10}$ =

S U M M A R Y

This chapter has reviewed basic arithmetic that will assist you to successfully implement dimensional analysis as a problem-solving method for medication dosage calculations. To assess your understanding and retention, complete the following practice problems.

Practice Problems for Chapter 1	**Arithmetic Review**
	(See pages 25–27 for answers)

Change the following Arabic numbers to Roman numerals.

1. 2 = II

2. 4 = IV

3. 5 = V

4. 14 = XIV

5. 19 =

Change the following Roman numerals to Arabic numbers.

6. VI   =

7. IX   =

8. XII =

9. XVII =

10. XIX =

Multiply the following fractions and reduce the answer to the lowest fractional term.

11. $\dfrac{3}{4} \times \dfrac{2}{5} =$

12. $\dfrac{2}{3} \times \dfrac{5}{8} =$

13. $\dfrac{1}{2} \times \dfrac{2}{3} =$

14. $\dfrac{7}{8} \times \dfrac{1}{3} =$

15. $\dfrac{4}{5} \times \dfrac{2}{7} =$

Divide the following fractions and reduce the answer to the lowest fractional term.

16. $\dfrac{1}{2} \div \dfrac{3}{4} =$

17. $\dfrac{1}{3} \div \dfrac{7}{8} =$

18. $\dfrac{1}{5} \div \dfrac{1}{2} =$

19. $\dfrac{4}{8} \div \dfrac{2}{3} =$

20. $\dfrac{1}{3} \div \dfrac{2}{3} =$

Multiply the following decimals.

21. $\begin{array}{r} 6.45 \\ \times\,\underline{1.36} \end{array}$

22. $\begin{array}{r} 3.14 \\ \times\,\underline{2.20} \end{array}$

23. $\begin{array}{r} 16.286 \\ \times\,\underline{\;0.125} \end{array}$

24. $\begin{array}{r} 1.2 \\ \times\underline{0.5} \end{array}$

25. $\begin{array}{r} 7.68 \\ \times\underline{0.05} \end{array}$

Divide the following decimals.

26. $0.5\overline{)1.25}$

27. $0.20\overline{)40.80}$

28. $0.125\overline{)0.25}$

29. $0.75\overline{)0.125}$

30. $0.5\overline{)7.30}$

(Practice Problems continue on page 18)

SECTION 1   Clinical Calculations

Convert the following fractions to decimals and round to the tenth.

31. $\dfrac{1}{2}$ =

32. $\dfrac{1}{3}$ =

33. $\dfrac{3}{4}$ =

34. $\dfrac{2}{3}$ =

35. $\dfrac{1}{8}$ =

Chapter 1 Post-Test: Arithmetic Review

Name _____ **Date** _____

Converting Between Arabic Numbers and Roman Numerals

1. 4 = _____

2. IX = _____

3. 16 = _____

4. XXV = _____

Multiplying and Dividing Fractions

5. $\dfrac{1}{8} \times \dfrac{1}{8}$ = _____

6. $\dfrac{2}{4} \times \dfrac{1}{2}$ = _____

7. $\dfrac{5}{6} \times \dfrac{3}{4}$ = _____

8. $\dfrac{1}{6} \div \dfrac{1}{3}$ = _____

9. $\dfrac{3}{4} \div \dfrac{7}{8}$ = _____

10. $\dfrac{1}{150} \div \dfrac{1}{2}$ = _____

Converting Fractions to Decimals

11. $\dfrac{1}{2}$ = _____

12. $\dfrac{3}{4}$ = _____

13. $\dfrac{7}{8}$ = _____

14. $\dfrac{2}{3}$ = _____

Multiplying and Dividing Decimals

15. 0.25×1.25 = _____

16. $0.125 \div 0.25$ = _____

17. 0.55×0.75 = _____

18. 1.5×0.25 = _____

19. $0.125 \div 0.5$ = _____

20. $0.525 \div 0.3$ = _____

ANSWER KEY FOR CHAPTER 1: ARITHMETIC REVIEW

Exercise 1.1 Arabic Numbers and Roman Numerals

1. 1	= I	
2. 1 + 1	= II	
3. 1 + 1 + 1	= III	
4. 5 − 1	= IV	
5. 5	= V	
6. 5 + 1	= VI	
7. 5 + 1 + 1	= VII	
8. 5 + 1 + 1 + 1	= VIII	
9. 10 − 1	= IX	
10. 10	= X	
11. 10 + 1	= XI	
12. 10 + 1 + 1	= XII	
13. 10 + 1 + 1 + 1	= XIII	
14. 10 + 5 − 1	= XIV	
15. 10 + 5	= XV	
16. 10 + 5 + 1	= XVI	
17. 10 + 5 + 1 + 1	= XVII	
18. 10 + 5 + 1 + 1 + 1	= XVIII	
19. 10 + 10 − 1	= XIX	
20. 10 + 10	= XX	
21. 50 − 10 + 1 + 1 + 1	= XLIII	
22. 10 + 10 + 5 − 1	= XXIV	
23. 50 + 5	= LV	
24. 10 + 10 + 10 + 1 + 1	= XXXII	
25. 100 + 1 + 1	= CII	
26. 100 + 50	= CL	
27. 50 + 10 + 10 + 5	= LXXV	
28. 100 − 10 + 1 + 1	= XCII	
29. 50 + 10 + 5 − 1	= LXIV	
30. 50 + 10 + 10 − 1	= LXIX	
31. 1 + 1	= 2	
32. 5 − 1	= 4	
33. 5 + 1	= 6	
34. 10	= 10	
35. 5 + 1 + 1 + 1	= 8	
36. 10 − 1 + 10	= 19	
37. 10 + 10	= 20	
38. 10 + 5 + 1 + 1 + 1	= 18	
39. 1	= 1	
40. 10 + 5	= 15	
41. 1 + 1 + 1	= 3	
42. 5	= 5	
43. 10 − 1	= 9	
44. 5 + 1 + 1	= 7	
45. 10 + 1	= 11	
46. 10 + 5 − 1	= 14	
47. 10 + 5 + 1	= 16	

48. 10 + 1 + 1	= 12	
49. 10 + 5 + 1 + 1	= 17	
50. 10 + 1 + 1 + 1	= 13	
51. 19	= XIX	
52. XII	= 12	
53. 7	= VII	
54. IX	= 9	
55. IV	= 4	
56. 11	= XI	
57. VIII	= 8	
58. 16	= XVI	
59. XX	= 20	
60. 5	= V	
61. I	= 1	
62. 18	= XVIII	
63. VI	= 6	
64. 2	= II	
65. III	= 3	
66. 10	= X	
67. XIII	= 13	
68. 14	= XIV	
69. XV	= 15	
70. 17	= XVII	

Exercise 1.2 Multiplying Fractions

1. $\dfrac{3}{4} \times \dfrac{5}{8} = \dfrac{3 \times 5 = 15}{4 \times 8 = 32} = \dfrac{15}{32}$

2. $\dfrac{1}{3} \times \dfrac{4}{9} = \dfrac{1 \times 4 = 4}{3 \times 9 = 27} = \dfrac{4}{27}$

3. $\dfrac{2}{3} \times \dfrac{4}{5} = \dfrac{2 \times 4 = 8}{3 \times 5 = 15} = \dfrac{8}{15}$

4. $\dfrac{3}{4} \times \dfrac{1}{2} = \dfrac{3 \times 1 = 3}{4 \times 2 = 8} = \dfrac{3}{8}$

5. $\dfrac{1}{8} \times \dfrac{4}{5} = \dfrac{1 \times 4 = 4\,(4) = 1}{8 \times 5 = 40(4) = 10} = \dfrac{1}{10}$

6. $\dfrac{2}{3} \times \dfrac{5}{8} = \dfrac{2 \times 5 = 10(2) = 5}{3 \times 8 = 24(2) = 12} = \dfrac{5}{12}$

7. $\dfrac{3}{8} \times \dfrac{2}{3} = \dfrac{3 \times 2 = 6\,(6) = 1}{8 \times 3 = 24(6) = 4} = \dfrac{1}{4}$

8. $\dfrac{4}{7} \times \dfrac{2}{4} = \dfrac{4 \times 2\ =\ 8\,(4)\ =\ 2}{7 \times 4\ =\ 28(4)\ =\ 7} = \dfrac{2}{7}$

9. $\dfrac{4}{5} \times \dfrac{1}{2} = \dfrac{4 \times 1\ =\ 4\,(2)\ =\ 2}{5 \times 2\ =\ 10(2)\ =\ 5} = \dfrac{2}{5}$

10. $\dfrac{1}{4} \times \dfrac{1}{8} = \dfrac{1 \times 1\ =\ 1}{4 \times 8\ =\ 32} = \dfrac{1}{32}$

Exercise 1.3 Dividing Fractions

1. $\dfrac{3}{4} \div \dfrac{2}{3} = \dfrac{3}{4} \times \dfrac{3}{2}$ or $\dfrac{3 \times 3 = 9}{4 \times 2 = 8} = 8\overline{)9}\;^{1\frac{1}{8}}\;\dfrac{8}{1} = 1\dfrac{1}{8}$

2. $\dfrac{1}{9} \div \dfrac{3}{9} = \dfrac{1}{9} \times \dfrac{9}{3}$ or $\dfrac{1 \times 9\ =\ 9\,(9)\ =\ 1}{9 \times 3\ =\ 27(9)\ =\ 3} = \dfrac{1}{3}$

3. $\dfrac{2}{3} \div \dfrac{1}{6} = \dfrac{2}{3} \times \dfrac{6}{1}$ or $\dfrac{2 \times 6 = 12}{3 \times 1 = 3} = 3\overline{)12}\;^{4}\;\dfrac{12}{\;} = 4$

4. $\dfrac{1}{5} \div \dfrac{4}{5} = \dfrac{1}{5} \times \dfrac{5}{4}$ or $\dfrac{1 \times 5\ =\ 5\,(5)\ =\ 1}{5 \times 4\ =\ 20(5)\ =\ 4} = \dfrac{1}{4}$

5. $\dfrac{3}{6} \div \dfrac{4}{8} = \dfrac{3}{6} \times \dfrac{8}{4}$ or $\dfrac{3 \times 8 = 24}{6 \times 4 = 24} = 24\overline{)24}\;^{1} = 1$

6. $\dfrac{5}{8} \div \dfrac{5}{8} = \dfrac{5}{8} \times \dfrac{8}{5}$ or $\dfrac{5 \times 8 = 40}{8 \times 5 = 40} = 40\overline{)40}\;^{1} = 1$

7. $\dfrac{1}{8} \div \dfrac{2}{3} = \dfrac{1}{8} \times \dfrac{3}{2}$ or $\dfrac{1 \times 3 = 3}{8 \times 2 = 16} = \dfrac{3}{16}$

8. $\dfrac{1}{5} \div \dfrac{1}{2} = \dfrac{1}{5} \times \dfrac{2}{1}$ or $\dfrac{1 \times 2 = 2}{5 \times 1 = 5} = \dfrac{2}{5}$

9. $\dfrac{1}{4} \div \dfrac{1}{2} = \dfrac{1 \times 2\ =\ 2(2)\ =\ 1}{4 \times 1\ =\ 4(2)\ =\ 2} = \dfrac{1}{2}$

10. $\dfrac{1}{6} \div \dfrac{1}{3} = \dfrac{1 \times 3\ =\ 3(3)\ =\ 1}{6 \times 1\ =\ 6(3)\ =\ 2} = \dfrac{1}{2}$

Exercise 1.4 Rounding Decimals

1. $0.75 = 0.8$
2. $0.88 = 0.9$
3. $0.44 = 0.4$
4. $0.23 = 0.2$
5. $0.67 = 0.7$
6. $0.27 = 0.3$
7. $0.98 = 1.0$
8. $0.92 = 0.9$
9. $0.64 = 0.6$
10. $0.250 = 0.3$

Exercise 1.5 Multiplying Decimals

1.   2.5 (1 decimal point)
   $\times$ 4.6 (1 decimal point)
     150
   1000
   1150
   11.50 (2 decimal points from the right to left)

2.   1.45 (2 decimal points)
   $\times$ 0.25 (2 decimal points)
     725
   2900
   0000
   3625
   0.3625 (4 decimal points from the right to left)

3.   3.9 (1 decimal point)
   $\times$ 0.8 (1 decimal point)
     312
   000
   312
   3.12 (2 decimal points from the right to left)

4.   2.56 (2 decimal points)
   $\times$ 0.45 (2 decimal points)
     1280
   10240
   00000
   11520
   1.1520 (4 decimal points from the right to left)

5. 10.65 (2 decimal points)
    × 0.05 (2 decimal points)
    ─────
    5325
    0000
    ─────
    5325
    0.5325 (4 decimal points from the right to left)

6.   1.98 (2 decimal points)
    × 3.10 (2 decimal points)
    ─────
    000
    1980
    59400
    ─────
    61380
    6.1380 (4 decimal points from the right to left)

7. 2.75 (2 decimal points)
    × 5.0 (1 decimal point)
    ─────
    000
    13750
    ─────
    13750
    13.750 (3 decimal points from the right to left)

8.   5.0 (1 decimal point)
    × 0.45 (2 decimal points)
    ─────
    250
    2000
    0000
    ─────
    2250
    2.250 (3 decimal points from the right to left)

9.   7.50 (2 decimal points)
    × 0.25 (2 decimal points)
    ─────
    3750
    15000
    00000
    ─────
    18750
    1.8750 (4 decimal points from the right to left)

10.   2.5 (1 decimal point)
    × 0.01 (2 decimal points)
    ─────
    25
    000
    0000
    ─────
    0025
    0.025 (3 decimal points from the right to left)

Exercise 1.6 Dividing Decimals

1. $3.4\overline{)9.6}$

    (Move decimal points one place to the right)

    Answer: 2.82 = 2.8

    ```
          2.82
    34)96.00
       68
       28 0
       27 2
          80
          68
          12
    ```

2. $0.25\overline{)12.50}$

    (Move decimal points two places to the right)

    Answer: 50. = 50

    ```
          50.
    25)1250.
       125
        00
    ```

3. $0.56\overline{)18.65}$

    (Move decimal points two places to the right)

    Answer: 33.30 = 33.3

    ```
          33.30
    56)1865.00
       168
       185
       168
        17 0
        16 8
           20
    ```

4. $0.3\overline{)0.192}$

    (Move decimal points one place to the right)

    Answer: 0.64 = 0.6

    ```
         .64
    3)01.92
      18
      12
      12
       0
    ```

5. $0.4\overline{)12.43}$

   (Move decimal points one place to the right)

   Answer: 31.075 = 31.1

   $$
   \begin{array}{r}
   31.075 \\
   4\overline{)124.300} \\
   \underline{12} \\
   04 \\
   \underline{4} \\
   0\,30 \\
   \underline{28} \\
   20 \\
   \underline{20} \\
   0
   \end{array}
   $$

6. $0.5\overline{)12.50}$

   (Move decimal points one place to the right)

   Answer: 25.0 = 25

   $$
   \begin{array}{r}
   25.0 \\
   5\overline{)125.0} \\
   \underline{10} \\
   25 \\
   \underline{25} \\
   0
   \end{array}
   $$

7. $0.125\overline{)0.25}$

   (Move decimal points three places to the right

   Answer: 2. = 2

   $$
   \begin{array}{r}
   2 \\
   125\overline{)250} \\
   \underline{250} \\
   0
   \end{array}
   $$

8. $0.08\overline{)0.085}$

   (Move decimal points two places to the right)

   Answer: 1.0625 = 1.1

   $$
   \begin{array}{r}
   1.0625 \\
   8\overline{)8.5000} \\
   \underline{8} \\
   50 \\
   \underline{48} \\
   20 \\
   \underline{16} \\
   40 \\
   \underline{40} \\
   0
   \end{array}
   $$

9. $1.5\overline{)22.5}$

   (Move decimal points one place to the right)

   Answer: 15. = 15

   $$
   \begin{array}{r}
   15. \\
   15.\overline{)225.} \\
   \underline{15} \\
   75 \\
   \underline{75}
   \end{array}
   $$

10. $5.5\overline{)16.5}$

    (Move decimal points one place to the right)

    Answer: 3. = 3

    $$
    \begin{array}{r}
    3. \\
    55.\overline{)165.} \\
    \underline{165}
    \end{array}
    $$

Exercise 1.7 Converting Fractions to Decimals

1. $\dfrac{1}{8}$ = 0.125

   Answer: 0.125

   $$
   \begin{array}{r}
   0.125 \\
   8\overline{)1.000} \\
   \underline{8} \\
   20 \\
   \underline{16} \\
   40 \\
   \underline{40} \\
   0
   \end{array}
   $$

2. $\dfrac{1}{4}$ = 0.25

   Answer: 0.25

   $$
   \begin{array}{r}
   .25 \\
   4\overline{)1.00} \\
   \underline{8} \\
   20 \\
   \underline{20} \\
   0
   \end{array}
   $$

3. $\frac{2}{5} = 0.4$

Answer: 0.4

$$\begin{array}{r} 0.4 \\ 5\overline{)2.0} \\ \underline{2\ 0} \\ 0 \end{array}$$

4. $\frac{3}{5} = 0.6$

Answer: 0.6

$$\begin{array}{r} 0.6 \\ 5\overline{)3.0} \\ \underline{3\ 0} \\ 0 \end{array}$$

5. $\frac{2}{3} = 0.66 = 0.7$

Answer: 0.66

$$\begin{array}{r} 0.66 \\ 3\overline{)2.00} \\ \underline{1\ 8} \\ 20 \\ \underline{18} \\ 2 \end{array}$$

6. $\frac{6}{8} = 0.75$

Answer: 0.75 = 0.8

$$\begin{array}{r} 0.75 \\ 8\overline{)6.00} \\ \underline{5\ 6} \\ 40 \\ \underline{40} \\ 0 \end{array}$$

7. $\frac{3}{8} = 0.375$

Answer: 0.375 = 0.38

$$\begin{array}{r} .375 \\ 8\overline{)3.00} \\ \underline{2\ 4} \\ 60 \\ \underline{56} \\ 40 \\ \underline{40} \\ 0 \end{array}$$

8. $\frac{1}{3} = 0.33$

Answer: 0.33 = 0.3

$$\begin{array}{r} 0.33 \\ 3\overline{)1.00} \\ \underline{9} \\ 10 \\ \underline{9} \\ 1 \end{array}$$

9. $\frac{3}{6} = 0.5$

Answer: 0.5

$$\begin{array}{r} 0.5 \\ 6\overline{)3.0} \\ \underline{3\ 0} \\ 0 \end{array}$$

10. $\frac{2}{10} = 0.2$

Answer: 0.2

$$\begin{array}{r} 0.2 \\ 10\overline{)2.0} \\ \underline{2\ 0} \\ 0 \end{array}$$

Practice Problems

1. II
2. IV
3. V
4. XIV
5. XIX
6. 6
7. 9
8. 12
9. 17
10. 19

11. $\frac{3 \times 2 = 6\,(2) = 3}{4 \times 5 = 20(2) = 10} = \frac{3}{10}$

12. $\frac{2 \times 5 = 10(2) = 5}{3 \times 8 = 24(2) = 12} = \frac{5}{12}$

13. $\frac{1 \times 2 = 2(2) = 1}{2 \times 3 = 6(2) = 3} = \frac{1}{3}$

14. $\dfrac{7 \times 1 = 7}{8 \times 3 = 24} = \dfrac{7}{24}$

15. $\dfrac{4 \times 2 = 8}{5 \times 7 = 35} = \dfrac{8}{35}$

16. $\dfrac{1}{2} \div \dfrac{3}{4} = \dfrac{1 \times 4 = 4(2) = 2}{2 \times 3 = 6(2) = 3} = \dfrac{2}{3}$

17. $\dfrac{1}{3} \div \dfrac{7}{8} = \dfrac{1 \times 8 = 8}{3 \times 7 = 21} = \dfrac{8}{21}$

18. $\dfrac{1}{5} \div \dfrac{1}{2} = \dfrac{1 \times 2 = 2}{5 \times 1 = 5} = \dfrac{2}{5}$

19. $\dfrac{4}{8} \div \dfrac{2}{3} = \dfrac{4 \times 3 = 12(4) = 3}{8 \times 2 = 16(4) = 4} = \dfrac{3}{4}$

20. $\dfrac{1}{3} \div \dfrac{2}{3} = \dfrac{1 \times 3 = 3(3) = 1}{3 \times 2 = 6(3) = 2} = \dfrac{1}{2}$

21.   6.45 (2 decimal points)
    × 1.36 (2 decimal points)
     3870
    19350
    64500
    87720
    8.7720 (4 decimal points from right to left)

22.   3.14 (2 decimal points)
    × 2.20 (2 decimal points)
     000
    6280
    62800
    69080
    6.9080 (4 decimal points from right to left)

23.   16.286 (3 decimal points)
    × 0.125 (3 decimal points)
     81430
    325720
    1628600
    2035750
    2.035750 (6 decimal points from right to left)

24.   1.2 (1 decimal point)
    ×0.5 (1 decimal point)
     60
    000
    060
    0.60 (2 decimal points from right to left)

25.   7.68 (2 decimal points)
    ×0.05 (2 decimal points)
     3840
    0000
    00000
    03840
    0.3840 (4 decimal points from right to left)

26. $0.5\overline{)1.25}$

    (Move decimal points one place to the right)

    Answer: 2.5

    $\begin{array}{r} 2.5 \\ 5\overline{)12.5} \\ \underline{10} \\ 2\,5 \\ \underline{2\,5} \\ 0 \end{array}$

27. $0.20\overline{)40.80}$

    (Move decimal points two places to the right)

    Answer: 204. = 204

    $\begin{array}{r} 204 \\ 20\overline{)4080} \\ \underline{40} \\ 080 \\ \underline{80} \\ 0 \end{array}$

28. $0.125\overline{)0.25}$

    (Move decimal points three places to the right)

    Answer: 2. = 2

    $\begin{array}{r} 2 \\ 125\overline{)250} \\ \underline{250} \\ 0 \end{array}$

29. $0.75\overline{)0.125}$

(Move decimal points two places to the right)

Answer: $0.166 = 0.17$

$$
\begin{array}{r}
.166 \\
75\overline{)12.500} \\
\underline{7\,5} \\
5\,00 \\
\underline{4\,50} \\
50
\end{array}
$$

30. $0.5\overline{)7.30}$

(Move decimal point one place to the right)

Answer: 14.6

$$
\begin{array}{r}
14.6 \\
5\overline{)73.0} \\
\underline{5} \\
23 \\
\underline{20} \\
3\,0 \\
\underline{3\,0} \\
0
\end{array}
$$

31. 0.5
32. 0.33 = 0.3
33. 0.75 = 0.8
34. 0.66 = 0.7
35. 0.125 = 0.13

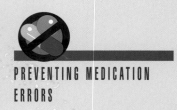

PREVENTING MEDICATION ERRORS

Medication calculation need not be difficult if you have a problem-solving method that is easy to understand and implement. In addition, you need to understand common equivalents and units of measurement to visualize all parts of a medication dosage calculation problem. Understanding common equivalents and units of measurement will assist you in preventing **medication errors** related to incorrect dosage.

This chapter will help you to understand the measurement systems used for medication administration. This knowledge is necessary to accurately implement the problem-solving method of dimensional analysis.

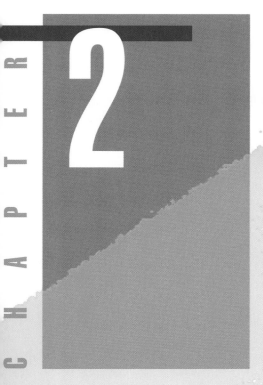

Systems of Measurement and Common Equivalents

Outline

SYSTEMS OF MEASUREMENT 30
THE METRIC SYSTEM 30
THE APOTHECARY SYSTEM 31
THE HOUSEHOLD SYSTEM 32
Temperature 33
COMMON EQUIVALENTS 34
Practice Problems for Chapter 2:
Systems of Measurement
and Common Equivalents 34
Post-Test for Chapter 2:
Systems of Measurement
and Common Equivalents 37
Answer Key for Chapter 2:
Systems of Measurement
and Common Equivalents 39

Objectives

After completing this chapter, you will be able to:

1. Identify measurements included in the metric, apothecary, and household systems.
2. Understand abbreviations used in the metric, apothecary, and household systems.

■ SYSTEMS OF MEASUREMENT

Three systems of measurement are used for medication dosage administration: the metric system, the apothecary system, and the household system. To be able to accurately administer medication, you must understand all three of these systems.

■ THE METRIC SYSTEM

The **metric system** is a decimal system of weights and measures based on units of ten in which gram, meter, and liter are the basic units of measurement. However, gram and liter are the only measurements from the metric system that are used in medication administration. The meter is a unit of distance, the gram (abbreviated g or gm) is a unit of weight, and the liter (abbreviated L) is a unit of volume.

The most frequently used metric units of *weight* and their equivalents are summarized in Box 2.1.

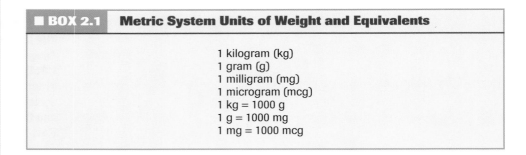

■ BOX 2.1	Metric System Units of Weight and Equivalents
	1 kilogram (kg) 1 gram (g) 1 milligram (mg) 1 microgram (mcg) 1 kg = 1000 g 1 g = 1000 mg 1 mg = 1000 mcg

Another way to understand the metric units of weight and their equivalents is to visualize the relationship between the measurements and equivalents displayed in Figure 2.1.

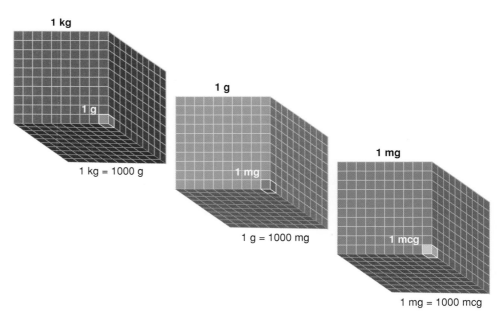

Figure 2.1.   Metric system units of weight and equivalents.

The most frequently used metric units for *volume* and their equivalents are summarized in Box 2.2.

Another way to understand the metric units of volume and their equivalents is to visualize the relationship between the measurements and equivalents displayed in Figure 2.2.

■ BOX 2.2	**Metric System Units of Volume and Equivalents**
	1 liter (L)
	1 milliliter (mL)
	1 cubic centimeter (cc)
	1 L = 1000 mL
	1 mL = 1 cc

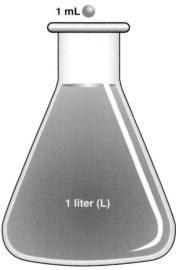

Figure 2.2. Metric system units of volume and equivalents.

■ THE APOTHECARY SYSTEM

The **apothecary system** is a system of measuring and weighing drugs and solutions in which fractions are used to identify parts of the unit of measure. The basic units of measurement in the apothecary system include weights and liquid volume. Although this may be replaced by the metric system, it is still necessary to understand it because some physicians continue to order medications using this system, and they also may include Roman numerals in the medication order.

The most frequently used measurements and equivalents within the apothecary system's units of *weight* are summarized in Box 2.3, and the most frequently used measurements and equivalents within the apothecary system's units of *volume* are summarized in Box 2.4. Figure 2.3 can help you visualize the equivalents for weight and volume.

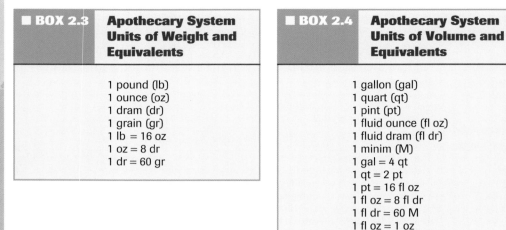

■ BOX 2.3	Apothecary System Units of Weight and Equivalents
	1 pound (lb)
	1 ounce (oz)
	1 dram (dr)
	1 grain (gr)
	1 lb = 16 oz
	1 oz = 8 dr
	1 dr = 60 gr

■ BOX 2.4	Apothecary System Units of Volume and Equivalents
	1 gallon (gal)
	1 quart (qt)
	1 pint (pt)
	1 fluid ounce (fl oz)
	1 fluid dram (fl dr)
	1 minim (M)
	1 gal = 4 qt
	1 qt = 2 pt
	1 pt = 16 fl oz
	1 fl oz = 8 fl dr
	1 fl dr = 60 M
	1 fl oz = 1 oz
	1 fl dr = 1 dr

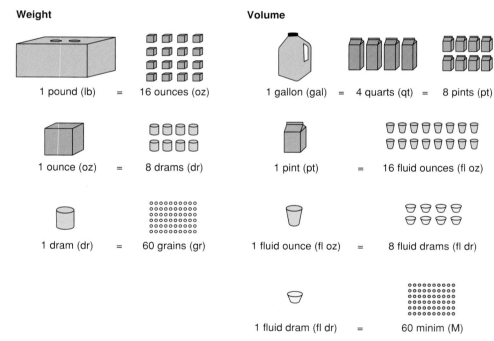

Weight

1 pound (lb) = 16 ounces (oz)

1 ounce (oz) = 8 drams (dr)

1 dram (dr) = 60 grains (gr)

Volume

1 gallon (gal) = 4 quarts (qt) = 8 pints (pt)

1 pint (pt) = 16 fluid ounces (fl oz)

1 fluid ounce (fl oz) = 8 fluid drams (fl dr)

1 fluid dram (fl dr) = 60 minim (M)

Figure 2.3. Apothecary system of equivalents for weight and volume. Please note that the figures are not shown to scale.

■ THE HOUSEHOLD SYSTEM

The use of household measurements is considered inaccurate because of the varying sizes of cups, glasses, and eating utensils, and this system generally has been replaced with the metric system. However, as patient care moves away from hospitals, which use the metric system, and into the community, it is once again necessary for the nurse to have an understanding of the household measurement system to be able to use and teach it to clients and families.

The most frequently used measurements and equivalents within the household measurement system are summarized in Box 2.5. Figure 2.4 can help you visualize the equivalents.

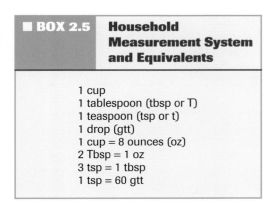

■ BOX 2.5 **Household Measurement System and Equivalents**

1 cup
1 tablespoon (tbsp or T)
1 teaspoon (tsp or t)
1 drop (gtt)
1 cup = 8 ounces (oz)
2 Tbsp = 1 oz
3 tsp = 1 tbsp
1 tsp = 60 gtt

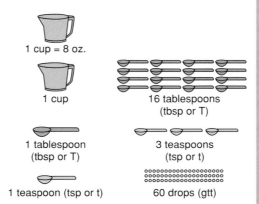

1 cup = 8 oz.

1 cup

16 tablespoons (tbsp or T)

1 tablespoon (tbsp or T)

3 teaspoons (tsp or t)

1 teaspoon (tsp or t)

60 drops (gtt)

Figure 2.4. Household measurement system and equivalents for volume. Please note that the figures are not shown to scale.

Temperature

Clients and families are required to monitor temperature changes associated with various medical conditions. Two thermometers may be used for monitoring temperature: a Fahrenheit thermometer or a Celsius thermometer. The nurse must be able to explain both of these systems of measurement when discharging clients and families.

The most frequently used measurements for Celsius and Fahrenheit are summarized in Figure 2.5.

Celsius	to	Fahrenheit
35.0		95.0
35.5		95.9
36.0		96.8
36.5		97.7
37.0		98.6
37.5		99.5
38.0		100.4
38.5		101.3
39.0		102.2
39.5		103.1
40.0		104.0
40.5		104.9
41.0		105.8
41.5		106.7
42.0		107.6

Figure 2.5. Conversion chart for Celsius to Fahrenheit.

Box 2.6 summarizes a method for converting between Celsius and Fahrenheit or Fahrenheit and Celsius. This easy method requires addition, subtraction, multiplication, or division.

■ BOX 2.6	**Temperature Conversion Method**

To convert from Fahrenheit to Celsius:
$^{\circ}C = (^{\circ}F - 32) \div 1.8$

To convert from Celsius to Fahrenheit:
$^{\circ}F = ^{\circ}C \times 1.8 + 32$

$^{\circ}C$ = temperature in degrees Celsius
$^{\circ}F$ = temperature in degrees Fahrenheit

■ COMMON EQUIVALENTS

Sometimes it is necessary to convert from one system to another to accurately administer medication. See Table 2.1 for approximate equivalents for weight and Table 2.2 for approximate equivalents for volume.

■ TABLE 2.1	**Approximate Equivalents for Weight**
METRIC	**APOTHECARY**
1 kg (1000 g)	2.2 lb
1 g (1000 mg)	15 gr
60 mg	1 gr

■ TABLE 2.2	**Approximate Equivalents for Volume**	
METRIC	**APOTHECARY**	**HOUSEHOLD**
4000 mL	1 gal (4 qt)	
1 L (1000 mL)	1 qt (2 pt)	
500 mL	1 pt (16 fl oz)	
240 mL	8 oz	1 cup (1 glass)
30 mL	1 oz (8 dr)	2 tbsp
15 mL	½ oz (4 dr)	1 tbsp (3 tsp)
5 mL	1 dr (60 M)	1 tsp (60 gtt)
1 mL (1 cc)	15 M	15 gtt
	1 M	1 gtt

S U M M A R Y

This chapter has reviewed the metric, apothecary, and household systems of measurement. To assess your understanding and retention of the systems of measurement, complete the following practice problems.

Practice Problems for Chapter 2	**Systems of Measurement and Common Equivalents**

(See page 39 for answers)

Write the correct abbreviation symbols for the following measurements from the metric system:

1. kilogram = Kg
2. gram = g

3. milligram = mg
4. microgram = mcg

PREVENTING MEDICATION ERRORS

Understanding the three systems of measurement will assist in preventing **medication errors.** Every nurse should have a chart that clearly identifies the conversions between the three systems of measurement to recheck answers for accuracy.

5. liter   = l

6. milliliter = ml

7. cubic centimeter = cc

Write the correct abbreviation symbols for the following measurements from the apothecary system:

8. pound = lb

9. ounce = oz

10. dram   = dr

11. grain   =

12. gallon =

13. quart   =

14. pint   =

15. fluid ounce =

16. fluid dram =

17. minim   =

Write the correct abbreviation symbols for the following measurements from the household system:

18. tablespoon =

19. teaspoon   =

20. drop   =

Identify the correct numerical values for the following measurements:

21. 1 kg = 2.2 lb

22. 1 kg = _____ g

23. 1 g   = 1000 mg

24. 1 mg = 1000 mcg

25. 1 g   = 15 gr

Identify the correct numerical values for the following temperatures:

26. 98.6°F   = _____ °C

27. 39°C   = _____ °F

28. 104.9°F = _____ °C

29. 36°C   = _____ °F

30. 101.3°F = _____ °C

Identify the correct numerical values for the following measurements:

31. 1 gr   = 60 mg

32. 1000 mg = 1 g

33. 1000 mL = 1 L = _____ qt

34. 500 mL = _____ pt

35. 240 mL = _____ oz

(Practice Problems continue on page 36)

36. 30 mL   = _____ oz   = _____ tbsp

37. 15 mL   = _____ oz   = _____ tsp

38. 5 mL   = _____ tsp

39. 1 mL   = _____ M   = _____ gtt

40. 1 mL   = _____ cc

41. 30 gtt = _____ M   = _____ mL

42. 4 tbsp = _____ oz   = _____ mL

43. 40°C   = _____ °F

44. 1 pt   = _____ fl oz = _____ mL

45. 2 qt   = _____ gal = _____ mL

46. 96.8°F = _____ °C

47. 2000 g = _____ kg   = _____ lb

48. gr xv   _____ g   = _____ mg

49. 37.5°C = _____ °F

50. 1 oz   = _____ dr   = _____ mL

51. 32 fl oz = _____ pt   = _____ mL

52. 39°C   = _____ °F

53. gr xxx = _____ g   = _____ mg

54. 240 mL = _____ oz   = _____ cup

55. 99.5°F = _____ °C

Chapter 2 Post-Test: Systems of Measurement and Common Equivalents

Name _____   **Date** _____

1. 2.2 lb   = _____ kg

2. 16 fl oz   = _____ pt

3. 1 tsp   = _____ mL

4. 15 gr   = _____ g

5. 1 oz   = _____ mL

6. 1000 mcg = _____ mg

7. 60 mg   = _____ gr

8. 1 pt   = _____ mL

9. 1 cc   = _____ mL

10. 1000 mg = _____ g

11. 1 L   = _____ mL

12. 4 qt   = _____ gal

13. 1 tbsp   = _____ tsp

14. 1 cup   = _____ oz

15. 8 oz   = _____ mL

16. 3 tsp   = _____ mL

17. 15 gtt   = _____ M

18. 1 dr   = _____ cc

19. 15 M   = _____ mL

20. 1000 g   = _____ kg

ANSWER KEY FOR CHAPTER 2: SYSTEMS OF MEASUREMENT AND COMMON EQUIVALENTS

Practice Problems

1. kilogram = kg
2. gram = g
3. milligram = mg
4. microgram = mcg
5. liter = L
6. milliliter = mL
7. cubic centimeter = cc
8. pound = lb
9. ounce = oz
10. dram = dr
11. grain = gr
12. gallon = gal
13. quart = qt
14. pint = pt
15. fluid ounce = fl oz
16. fluid dram = fl dr
17. minim = M
18. tablespoon = tbsp
19. teaspoon = tsp
20. drop = gtt
21. 1 kg = 2.2 lb
22. 1 kg = 1000 g
23. 1 g = 1000 mg
24. 1 mg = 1000 mcg
25. 1 g = 15 gr
26. 98.6°F = 37°C
27. 39°C = 102.2°F
28. 104.9°F = 40.5°C

29. 36°C = 96.8°F
30. 101.3°F = 38.5°C
31. 1 gr = 60 mg
32. 1000 mg = 1 g
33. 1000 mL = 1 L = 1 qt
34. 500 mL = 1 pt
35. 240 mL = 8 oz
36. 30 mL = 1 oz = 2 tbsp
37. 15 mL = ½ oz = 3 tsp
38. 5 mL = 1 tsp
39. 1 mL = 15 M = 15 gtt
40. 1 mL = 1 cc
41. 30 gtt = 30 M = 2 mL
42. 4 tbsp = 2 oz = 60 mL
43. 40°C = 104°F
44. 1 pt = 16 fl oz = 500 mL
45. 2 qt = ½ gal = 2000 mL
46. 96.8°F = 36°C
47. 2000 g = 2 kg = 4.4 lb
48. gr xv = 1 g = 1000 mg
49. 37.5°C = 99.5°F
50. 1 oz = 8 dr = 30 mL
51. 32 fl oz = 2 pt = 1000 mL
52. 39°C = 102.2°F
53. gr xxx = 2 g = 1800 mg
54. 240 mL = 8 oz = 1 cup
55. 99.5°F = 37.5°C

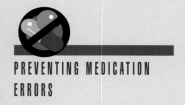

PREVENTING MEDICATION ERRORS

Dimensional analysis provides a systematic, straight-forward way to set up problems and to organize and evaluate data. It is not only easy to learn, but also can reduce **medication errors** when mathematical conversion is required.

Dimensional analysis assists with preventing medication errors by allowing you to visualize all parts of the medication problem and to critically think your way through the problem.

This chapter introduces you to dimensional analysis with a step-by-step explanation of this problem-solving method. The chapter also provides the opportunity to practice solving problems that involve common equivalents.

3

Solving Problems Using Dimensional Analysis

Outline

**TERMS USED
IN DIMENSIONAL ANALYSIS**   42
**THE FIVE STEPS
OF DIMENSIONAL ANALYSIS**   42
Exercise 3.1: Dimensional Analysis   46
**Practice Problems for Chapter 3:
Solving Problems Using
Dimensional Analysis**   49
**Post-Test for Chapter 3:
Solving Problems Using
Dimensional Analysis**   51
**Answer Key for Chapter 3:
Solving Problems Using
Dimensional Analysis**   53

Objectives

After completing this chapter, you will be able to:

1. Define the terms used in dimensional analysis.
2. Explain the step-by-step problem-solving method of dimensional analysis.
3. Solve problems involving common equivalents using dimensional analysis as a problem-solving method.

■ TERMS USED IN DIMENSIONAL ANALYSIS

Dimensional analysis is a problem-solving method that can be used whenever two quantities are directly proportional to each other and one quantity must be converted to the other by using a common equivalent, conversion factor, or conversion relation. All medication dosage calculation problems can be solved by dimensional analysis.

It is important to understand the following four terms that provide the basis for dimensional analysis.

- **Given quantity:** the beginning point of the problem
- **Wanted quantity:** the answer to the problem
- **Unit path:** the series of conversions necessary to achieve the answer to the problem
- **Conversion factors:** equivalents necessary to convert between systems of measurement and to allow unwanted units to be canceled from the problem
  Each conversion factor is a ratio of units that equals 1.

Dimensional analysis also uses the same terms as fractions: numerators and denominators.

- *Numerator* = the top portion of the problem
- *Denominator* = the bottom portion of the problem

Some problems will have a given quantity and a wanted quantity that contain only numerators. Other problems will have a given quantity and a wanted quantity that contain both a numerator and a denominator. This chapter contains only problems with numerators as the given quantity and the wanted quantity.

Once the beginning point in the problem is identified, then a series of conversions necessary to achieve the answer is established that leads to the problem's solution.

Below is an example of the problem-solving method, showing the placement of basic terms used in dimensional analysis.

Unit Path

Given Quantity	Conversion Factor for Given Quantity	Conversion Factor for Wanted Quantity	Conversion Computation	Wanted Quantity
1 liter (L)	1000 mL	1 oz	$1 \times 1000 \times 1$	$\dfrac{1000}{30} = 33.3$ oz
	1 liter (L)	30 mL	1×30	

■ THE FIVE STEPS OF DIMENSIONAL ANALYSIS

Once the given quantity is identified, the unit path leading to the wanted quantity is established. The problem-solving method of dimensional analysis uses the following five steps.

1. Identify the *given quantity* in the problem.
2. Identify the *wanted quantity* in the problem.

3. Establish the *unit path* from the given quantity to the wanted quantity using equivalents as *conversion factors*.
4. Set up the conversion factors to permit cancellation of unwanted units. Carefully choose each conversion factor and ensure that it is correctly placed in the numerator or denominator portion of the problem to allow the unwanted units to be canceled from the problem.
5. Multiply the numerators, multiply the denominators, and divide the product of the numerators by the product of the denominators to provide the numerical value of the wanted quantity.

The following examples use the five steps to solve problems using dimensional analysis.

EXAMPLE 3.1

▷ **1 liter (L) equals how many ounces (oz)?**

STEP 1 Identify the *given quantity* in the problem.

Unit Path

Given Quantity	Conversion Factor for Given Quantity	Conversion Factor for Wanted Quantity	Conversion Computation		Wanted Quantity
1 liter (L)				=	

▶▶▶ *The given quantity is* 1 L.

STEP 2 Identify the *wanted quantity* in the problem.

Unit Path

Given Quantity	Conversion Factor for Given Quantity	Conversion Factor for Wanted Quantity	Conversion Computation		Wanted Quantity
1 liter (L)				= oz	

▶▶▶ *The wanted quantity is the number of* ounces *(oz) in 1 L.*

STEP 3 Establish the *unit path* from the given quantity to the wanted quantity. You must determine what conversion factors are needed to convert the given quantity to the wanted quantity.

▶▶▶ *Given quantity: 1 L = 1000 mL*
Wanted quantity: 1 oz = 30 mL

(Example continues on page 44)

STEP 4 Write the unit path for the problem so that each unit cancels out the preceding unit until all unwanted units are canceled from the problem except the wanted quantity.

> The wanted quantity must be within the numerator portion of the problem to identify that the problem is set up correctly.

Unit Path

Given Quantity	Conversion Factor for Given Quantity	Conversion Factor for Wanted Quantity	Conversion Computation	Wanted Quantity
1 liter (L)	1000 mL	1 oz		
	1 liter (L)	30 mL		= oz

Unit Path

Given Quantity	Conversion Factor for Given Quantity	Conversion Factor for Wanted Quantity	Conversion Computation	Wanted Quantity
1 liter (L)	1000 mL	1 oz		
	1 liter (L)	30 mL		= oz

STEP 5 After the unwanted units are canceled from the problem, only the numerical values remain. Multiply the numerators, multiply the denominators, and divide the product of the numerators by the product of the denominators to provide the numerical value for the wanted quantity.

> One (1) times (×) any number equals that number, therefore 1s may be automatically canceled from the problem. Other factors that can be canceled from the problem include like numerical values in the numerator and denominator portion of the problem and the same number of zeroes in the numerator and denominator portion of the problem.

Unit Path

Given Quantity	Conversion Factor for Given Quantity	Conversion Factor for Wanted Quantity	Conversion Computation		Wanted Quantity
1 liter (L)	1000 mL	1 oz	1000×1	1000	
	1 liter (L)	30 mL	1×30	30	= 33.3 oz

▶ ▶ ▶ *33.3 oz is the wanted quantity and the answer to the problem.*

EXAMPLE 3.2

▶ **One gallon (gal) equals how many milliliters (mL)?**

STEP 1 Identify the given quantity in the problem.

$$\frac{1\ \text{gal}}{} =$$

▶ ▶ ▶ *The given quantity is 1 gal.*

STEP 2 Identify the wanted quantity in the problem.

$$\frac{1\ \text{gal}}{} = \text{mL}$$

▶ ▶ ▶ *The wanted quantity is the number of milliliters (mL) in 1 gal.*

STEP 3 Establish the unit path from the given quantity to the wanted quantity by selecting the equivalents that will be used as conversion factors.

▶ ▶ ▶ *Given quantity: 1 gal = 4 quarts (qt); 1 qt = 1 L*
Wanted quantity: 1 L = 1000 mL

STEP 4 Write the unit path for the problem so that each unit cancels out the preceding unit until all unwanted units are canceled from the problem except the wanted quantity.

$$\frac{1\ \cancel{\text{gal}}}{} \left| \frac{4\ \text{qt}}{1\ \cancel{\text{gal}}} \right| \frac{1\ \cancel{\text{L}}}{1\ \cancel{\text{qt}}} \left| \frac{1000\ \text{mL}}{1\ \cancel{\text{L}}} \right. = \quad \text{mL}$$

STEP 5 After the unwanted units are canceled from the problem, only the numerical values remain. Multiply the numerators, multiply the denominators, and divide the product of the numerators by the product of the denominators to provide the numerical value for the wanted quantity.

$$\frac{\cancel{1\ \text{gal}}}{} \left| \frac{4\ \text{qt}}{\cancel{1\ \text{gal}}} \right| \frac{\cancel{1\ \text{L}}}{\cancel{1\ \text{qt}}} \left| \frac{1000\ \text{mL}}{1\ \cancel{\text{L}}} \right| \frac{4 \times 1000}{1} = 4000\ \text{mL}$$

▶ ▶ ▶ *4000 mL is the wanted quantity and the answer to the problem.*

Exercise 3.1   **Dimensional Analysis**
(See pages 53–54 for answers)

Use dimensional analysis to change the following units of measurement.

1. Problem: 4 mg = How many g?

   Given quantity   =

   Wanted quantity   =

$$\frac{4 \text{ mg}}{} \left| \frac{1 \text{ g}}{1000 \text{ mg}} \right. \qquad\qquad = \qquad \text{g}$$

2. Problem: 5000 g = How many kg?

   Given quantity   =

   Wanted quantity   =

$$\frac{5000 \text{ g}}{} \left| \frac{1 \text{ kg}}{1000 \text{ g}} \right. \qquad\qquad = \qquad \text{kg}$$

3. Problem: 0.3 L = How many cc?

   Given quantity   =

   Wanted quantity   =

$$\frac{0.3 \text{ L}}{} \left| \right. \qquad\qquad = \qquad \text{cc}$$

4. Problem: 10 cc = How many mL?

   Given quantity   =

   Wanted quantity   =

$$\frac{10 \text{ cc}}{} \left| \frac{1 \text{ ml}}{1 \text{ cc}} \right. \qquad\qquad = 10 \text{ mL}$$

5. Problem: 120 lb = How many kg?

   Given quantity   =

   Wanted quantity   =

$$\frac{120 \text{ lb}}{} \left| \frac{1 \text{ kg}}{2.2 \text{ lb}} \right. \qquad\qquad = \qquad \text{kg}$$

6. Problem: 5 gr = How many mg?

Given quantity =

Wanted quantity =

$$\frac{5 \text{ gr} \quad | \quad 60 \text{ mg}}{| \quad 1 \text{ gr}} = \quad \text{mg}$$

7. Problem: 2 g = How many gr?

Given quantity = 2g | 160 mg | grain

Wanted quantity =

$$\frac{2 \text{ g} \quad | \quad 1000 \text{ mg} \quad | \quad 1 \text{ gr}}{| \quad 1 \text{ g} \quad | \quad 60 \text{ mg}} = \quad \text{gr}$$

8. Problem: 5 fl dr = How many mL?

Given quantity =

Wanted quantity =

$$\frac{5 \text{ fl dr} \quad |}{|} = \quad \text{mL}$$

9. Problem: 8 fl dr = How many fl oz?

Given quantity =

Wanted quantity =

$$\frac{8 \text{ fl dr} \quad |}{|} = \quad \text{fl oz}$$

10. Problem: 10 M = How many fl dr?

Given quantity =

Wanted quantity =

$$\frac{10 \text{ M} \quad | \quad \text{IML} \quad | \quad 1}{| \quad 15 \text{M} \quad | \quad 5 \text{ ml}} \quad \frac{10}{75} = 0.13 \text{ fl dr}$$

11. Problem: 35 kg = How many lb?

Given quantity =

Wanted quantity =

$$\frac{35 \text{ kg} \quad | \quad 2.2 \text{ lb}}{| \quad 1 \text{ kg}} = \quad \text{lb}$$

(Exercise continues on page 48)

12. Problem: 10 mL = How many tsp?

   Given quantity   =

   Wanted quantity   =

   $$\frac{10\ \text{mL}\ \big|}{\big|} \rule{6cm}{0.4pt} =\quad \text{tsp}$$

13. Problem: 30 mL = How many tbsp?

   Given quantity   =

   Wanted quantity   =

   $$\frac{30\ \text{mL}\ \big|}{\big|} \rule{6cm}{0.4pt} =\quad \text{tbsp}$$

14. Problem: 0.25 g = How many mg?

   Given quantity   =

   Wanted quantity   =

   $$\frac{0.25\ \text{g}\ \big|}{\big|} \rule{6cm}{0.4pt} =\quad \text{mg}$$

15. Problem: 350 mcg = How many mg?

   Given quantity   =

   Wanted quantity   =

   $$\frac{350\ \text{mcg}\ \big|}{\big|} \rule{6cm}{0.4pt} =\quad \text{mg}$$

16. Problem: 0.75 L = How many mL?

   Given quantity   =

   Wanted quantity   =

   $$\frac{0.75\ \text{L}\ \big|}{\big|} \rule{6cm}{0.4pt} =\quad \text{mL}$$

17. Problem: 3 hr = How many minutes?

   Given quantity   =

   Wanted quantity   =

   $$\frac{3\ \text{hr}\ \big|}{\big|} \rule{6cm}{0.4pt} =\quad \text{min}$$

18. Problem: 3.5 mL = How many M?

    Given quantity   =

    Wanted quantity   =

    $$\dfrac{3.5\ \text{mL}\ \big|}{} = \quad \text{M}$$

19. Problem: 500 mcg = How many mg?

    Given quantity   =

    Wanted quantity   =

    $$\dfrac{500\ \text{mcg}\ \big|}{} = \quad \text{mg}$$

20. Problem: 225 M = How many tsp?

    Given quantity   =

    Wanted quantity   =

    $$\dfrac{225\ \text{M}\ \big|}{} = \quad \text{tsp}$$

S U M M A R Y

This chapter has introduced you to dimensional analysis with a step-by-step explanation and an opportunity to practice solving problems involving common equivalents. To demonstrate your understanding of dimensional analysis and conversions between systems of measurement, complete the following practice problems.

Practice Problems for Chapter 3	**Solving Problems Using Dimensional Analysis**

(See pages 55–56 for answers)

1. Problem: $\frac{3}{4}$ mL   = How many M?

2. Problem: gtt XV = How many M?

3. Problem: $\frac{5}{6}$ gr   = How many mg?

4. Problem: How many mL in 3 oz?

5. Problem: 0.5 mg = How many mcg?

6. Problem: 35 gtt = How many mL?

7. Problem: How many cc in 3 qt?

(Practice Problems continue on page 50)

8. Problem: 4 gal   = How many qt?

9. Problem: 1.5 cup   = How many cc?

10. Problem: 24 oz   = How many cups?

11. Problem: 132 lb   = How many kg?

12. Problem: 70 kg   = How many lb?

13. Problem: 750 mcg   = How many mg?

14. Problem: 0.5 L   = How many mL?

15. Problem: 1800 g   = How many kg?

16. Problem: 39°C   = How many °F?

17. Problem: 180 mL   = How many oz?

18. Problem: 6 dr   = How many mL?

19. Problem: 0.125 mg = How many mcg?

20. Problem: 98.8°F   = How many °C?

Chapter 3 Post-Test: Solving Problems Using Dimensional Analysis

Name _____ **Date** _____

Use dimensional analysis to solve the following conversion problems:

 1. 2045 g = How many lb?

 2. 1/150 gr = How many mg?

 3. 0.004 g = How many mcg?

 4. 6 tsp = How many dr?

 5. 0.5 L = How many pt?

 6. How many L in 250 oz?

 7. How many tbsp in 30 cc?

 8. How many minims in 60 cc?

 9. How many g in 45 gr?

10. How many oz in 1800 g?

11. 300 mg = How many gr?

12. How many mg in gr 1/4?

13. 20 mL = How many M?

14. How many mcg in 0.75 mg?

15. 94°F = How many °C?

16. How many lb in 84 kg?

17. 1/300 gr = How many mg?

18. 100°F = How many °C?

19. How many gr in 30 mg?

20. 39.2°C = How many °F?

ANSWER KEY FOR CHAPTER 3: SOLVING PROBLEMS USING DIMENSIONAL ANALYSIS

Exercise 3.1 **Dimensional Analysis**

1. Problem: 4 mg = How many g?
   Given quantity   = 4 mg
   Wanted quantity   = g
   Conversion factor   = 1 g = 1000 mg

4 mg	1 ⓖ	4 × 1	4	= 0.004 g
	1000 mg	1000	1000	

2. Problem: 5000 g = How many kg?
   Given quantity   = 5000 g
   Wanted quantity   = kg
   Conversion factor   = 1 kg = 1000 g

5000 g	1 ⓚⓖ	5 × 1	5	= 5 kg
	1000 g	1	1	

3. Problem: 0.3 L = How many cc?
   Given quantity   = 0.3 L
   Wanted quantity   = cc
   Conversion factor   = 1 L = 1000 cc

0.3 Ł	1000 ⓒⓒ	0.3 × 1000	300	= 300 cc
	1 Ł	1	1	

4. Problem: 10 cc = How many mL?
   Given quantity   = 10 cc
   Wanted quantity   = mL
   Conversion factor   = 1 cc = 1 mL

10 cc	1 ⓜⓁ	10 × 1	10	= 10 mL
	1 cc	1	1	

5. Problem: 120 lb = How many kg?
   Given quantity   = 120 lb
   Wanted quantity   = kg
   Conversion factor   = 2.2 lb = 1 kg

120 ℔	1 ⓚⓖ	120 × 1	120	= 54.5 kg
	2.2 ℔	2.2	2.2	

6. Problem: 5 gr = How many mg?
   Given quantity   = 5 gr
   Wanted quantity   = mg
   Conversion factor   = 1 gr = 60 mg

5 gr	60 ⓜⓖ	5 × 60	300	= 300 mg
	1 gr	1	1	

7. Problem: 2 g = How many gr?
   Given quantity   = 2 g
   Wanted quantity   = gr
   Conversion factor   = 1 g = 15 gr

2 g	15 ⓖⓡ	2 × 15	30	= 30 gr
	1 g	1	1	

8. Problem: 5 fl dr = How many mL?
   Given quantity   = 5 fl dr
   Wanted quantity   = mL
   Conversion factor   = 1 fl dr = 5 mL

5 fl dr	5 ⓜⓁ	5 × 5	25	= 25 mL
	1 fl dr	1	1	

9. Problem: 8 fl dr = How many fl oz?
   Given quantity   = 8 fl dr
   Wanted quantity   = fl oz
   Conversion factor   = 1 fl dr = 5 mL
   Conversion factor   = 1 fl oz = 30 mL

8 fl dr	5 mŁ	1 ⓕⓁⓞⓩ	8 × 5 × 1	40	= 1.3 fl oz
	1 fl dr	30 mŁ	1 × 30	30	

10. Problem: 10 M = How many fl dr?
    Given quantity   = M
    Wanted quantity   = fl dr
    Conversion factor   = 1 mL = 15 M
    Conversion factor   = 1 fl dr = 5 mL

10 M	1 mŁ	1 ⓕⓁⓓⓡ	10 × 1 × 1	10	= 0.13 fl dr
	15 M	5 mŁ	15 × 5	75	

11. Problem: 35 kg = How many lb?
    Given quantity   = 35 kg
    Wanted quantity   = lb
    Conversion factor = 1 kg = 2.2 lb

35 kg	2.2 (lb)	35 × 2.2	77 = 77 lb
	1 kg	1	1

12. Problem: 10 mL = How many tsp?
    Given quantity   = 10 mL
    Wanted quantity   = tsp
    Conversion factor = 1 tsp = 5 mL

10 mL	1 (tsp)	10 × 1	10 = 2 tsp
	5 mL	5	5

13. Problem: 30 mL = How many tbsp?
    Given quantity   = 30 mL
    Wanted quantity   = tbsp
    Conversion factor = 1 tbsp = 15 mL

30 mL	1 (tbsp)	30 × 1	30 = 2 tbsp
	15 mL	15	15

14. Problem: 0.25 g = How many mg?
    Given quantity   = 0.25 g
    Wanted quantity   = mg
    Conversion factor = 1 g = 1000 mg

0.25 g	1000 (mg)	0.25 × 1000	250 = 250 mg
	1 g	1	1

15. Problem: 350 mcg = How many mg?
    Given quantity   = 350 mcg
    Wanted quantity   = mg
    Conversion factor = 1 mg = 1000 mcg

350 mcg	1 (mg)	350 × 1	350 = 0.35 mg
	1000 mcg	1000	1000

16. Problem: 0.75 L = How many mL?
    Given quantity   = 0.75 L
    Wanted quantity   = mL
    Conversion factor = 1 L = 1000 mL

0.75 L	1000 (mL)	0.75 × 1000	750 = 750 mL
	1 L	1	1

17. Problem: 3 hr = How many minutes?
    Given quantity   = 3 hr
    Wanted quantity   = minutes
    Conversion factor = 1 hr = 60 min

3 hr	60 (min)	3 × 60	180 = 180 min
	1 hr	1	1

18. Problem: 3.5 mL = How many M?
    Given quantity   = 3.5 mL
    Wanted quantity   = M
    Conversion factor = 1 mL = 15 M

3.5 mL	15 (M)	3.5 × 15	52.5 = 52.5 M
	1 mL	1	1

19. Problem: 500 mcg = How many mg?
    Given quantity   = 500 mcg
    Wanted quantity   = mg
    Conversion factor = 1 mg = 1000 mcg

500 mcg	1 (mg)	500 × 1	500 = 0.5 mg
	1000 mcg	1000	1000

20. Problem: 225 M = How many tsp?
    Given quantity   = 225 M
    Wanted quantity   = tsp
    Conversion factor = 1 mL = 15 M
    Conversion factor = 1 tsp = 5 mL

225 M	1 mL	1 (tsp)	225 × 1 × 1	225 = 3 tsp
	15 M	5 mL	15 × 5	75

Practice Problems

1. Problem: $\frac{3}{4}$ mL = How many M?
   Given quantity   = $\frac{3}{4}$ mL
   Wanted quantity   = M
   Conversion factor = 1 mL = 15 M

$$\frac{\frac{3}{4}\,\text{mL}}{1\,\text{mL}} \left|\, \frac{15\,\text{(M)}}{1} \,\right|\, \frac{\frac{3}{4} \times 15}{1} \left|\, \frac{\frac{3}{4} \times \frac{15}{1}}{1} \,\right|\, \frac{45}{4} = 11.25\ \text{M}$$

2. Problem: gtt XV = How many M?
   Given quantity   = 15 gtt
   Wanted quantity   = M
   Conversion factor = 1 gtt = 1 M

$$\frac{15\ \text{gtt}}{1\ \text{gtt}} \left|\, \frac{1\ \text{(M)}}{} \,\right|\, 15 = 15\ \text{M}$$

3. Problem: $\frac{5}{6}$ gr = How many mg?
   Given quantity   = $\frac{5}{6}$ gr
   Wanted quantity   = mg
   Conversion factor = 1 gr = 60 mg

$$\frac{\frac{5}{6}\ \text{gr}}{1\ \text{gr}} \left|\, \frac{60\ \text{(mg)}}{1} \,\right|\, \frac{\frac{5}{6} \times 60}{1} \left|\, \frac{\frac{5}{6} \times \frac{60}{1}}{1} \,\right|\, \frac{300}{6} \,\right|\, 50 = 50\ \text{mg}$$

4. Problem: How many mL in 3 oz?
   Given quantity   = 3 oz
   Wanted quantity   = mL
   Conversion factor = 1 oz = 30 mL

$$\frac{3\ \text{oz}}{1\ \text{oz}} \left|\, \frac{30\ \text{(mL)}}{1} \,\right|\, \frac{3 \times 30}{1} \,\right|\, 90 = 90\ \text{mL}$$

5. Problem: 0.5 mg = How many mcg?
   Given quantity   = 0.5 mg
   Wanted quantity   = mcg
   Conversion factor = 1 mg = 1000 mcg

$$\frac{0.5\ \text{mg}}{1\ \text{mg}} \left|\, \frac{1000\ \text{(mcg)}}{1} \,\right|\, \frac{0.5 \times 1000}{1} \,\right|\, 500 = 500\ \text{mcg}$$

6. Problem: 35 gtt = How many mL?
   Given quantity   = 35 gtt
   Wanted quantity   = mL
   Conversion factor = 1 gtt = 1 M
   Conversion factor = 15 M = 1 mL

$$\frac{35\ \text{gtt}}{1\ \text{gtt}} \left|\, \frac{1\ \text{M}}{15\ \text{M}} \,\right|\, \frac{1\ \text{(mL)}}{} \,\right|\, \frac{35 \times 1 \times 1}{1 \times 15} \,\right|\, \frac{35}{15} = 2.3\ \text{mL}$$

7. Problem: How many cc in 3 qt?
   Given quantity   = 3 qt
   Wanted quantity   = cc
   Conversion factor = 1 qt = 1000 mL
   Conversion factor = 1 cc = 1 mL

$$\frac{3\ \text{qt}}{1\ \text{qt}} \left|\, \frac{1000\ \text{mL}}{1\ \text{mL}} \,\right|\, \frac{1\ \text{(cc)}}{} \,\right|\, \frac{3 \times 1000 \times 1}{1 \times 1} \,\right|\, \frac{3000}{1} = 3000\ \text{cc}$$

8. Problem: 4 gal = How many qt?
   Given quantity   = 4 gal
   Wanted quantity   = qt
   Conversion factor = 1 gal = 4 qt

$$\frac{4\ \text{gal}}{1\ \text{gal}} \left|\, \frac{4\ \text{(qt)}}{1} \,\right|\, \frac{4 \times 4}{1} \,\right|\, 16 = 16\ \text{qt}$$

9. Problem: 1.5 cup = How many cc?
   Given quantity   = 1.5 cup
   Wanted quantity   = cc
   Conversion factor = 1 cup = 240 cc

$$\frac{1.5\ \text{cup}}{1\ \text{cup}} \left|\, \frac{240\ \text{(cc)}}{1} \,\right|\, \frac{1.5 \times 240}{1} \,\right|\, \frac{360}{1} = 360\ \text{cc}$$

10. Problem: 24 oz = How many cups?
    Given quantity   = 24 oz
    Wanted quantity   = cups
    Conversion factor = 1 cup = 8 oz

$$\frac{24\ \text{oz}}{8\ \text{oz}} \left|\, \frac{1\ \text{(cup)}}{8} \,\right|\, \frac{24 \times 1}{8} \,\right|\, \frac{24}{8} = 3\ \text{cups}$$

11. Problem: 132 lb   = How many kg?
    Given quantity   = 132 lb
    Wanted quantity   = kg
    Conversion factor = 2.2 lb = 1 kg

132 lb	1 (kg)	132 × 1	132	= 60 kg
	2.2 lb	2.2	2.2	

12. Problem: 70 kg   = How many lb?
    Given quantity   = 70 kg
    Wanted quantity   = lb
    Conversion factor = 1 kg = 2.2 lb

70 kg	2.2 (lb)	70 × 2.2	154	= 154 lb
	1 kg	1	1	

13. Problem: 750 mcg = How many mg?
    Given quantity   = 750 mcg
    Wanted quantity   = mg
    Conversion factor = 1000 mcg = 1 ml

750 mcg	1 (mg)	75 × 1	75	= 0.75 mg
	1000 mcg	100	100	

14. Problem: 0.5 L   = How many mL?
    Given quantity   = 0.5 L
    Wanted quantity   = mL
    Conversion factor = 1 L = 1000 mL

0.5 L	1000 (mL)	0.5 × 1000	500	= 500 mL
	1 L	1	1	

15. Problem: 1800 g   = How many kg?
    Given quantity   = 1800 g
    Wanted quantity   = kg
    Conversion factor = 1000 g = 1 kg

1800 g	1 (kg)	18 × 1	18	= 1.8 kg
	1000 g	10	10	

16. °F = 39°C × 1.8 + 32 = 102.2°F

17. Problem: 180 mL   = How many oz?
    Given quantity   = 180 mL
    Wanted quantity   = oz
    Conversion factor = 30 mL = 1 oz

180 mL	1 (oz)	18 × 1	18	= 6 oz
	30 mL	3	3	

18. Problem: 6 dr   = How many mL?
    Given quantity   = 6 dr
    Wanted quantity   = mL
    Conversion factor = 1 dr = 5 mL

6 dr	5 (mL)	6 × 5	30	= 30 mL
	1 dr	1	1	

19. Problem: 0.125 mg = How many mcg?
    Given quantity   = 0.125 mg
    Wanted quantity   = mcg
    Conversion factor = 1 mg = 1000 mcg

0.125 mg	1000 (mcg)	0.125 × 1000	125	= 125 mcg
	1 mg	1	1	

20. °C = 98.8°F − 32 ÷ 1.8 = 37.1°C

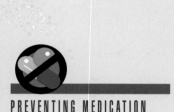

PREVENTING MEDICATION ERRORS

For accurate administration of medication, the five rights of medication administration form the foundation of communication between the person writing the medication order and the person reading the medication order.

The physician or nurse practitioner writes a medication order using the five rights, and the nurse administers the medication to the patient based on the five rights. There may be a slight variation in the way each person writes a medication order, but information pertaining to the five rights should be included in the medication order to ensure safe administration by the nurse and the prevention of **medication errors.**

To calculate the change from a one-factor-given quantity to a one-factor-wanted quantity using dimensional analysis, it is necessary to have a clear understanding of the five rights of medication administration. This chapter teaches you to interpret medication orders correctly and to calculate medication problems accurately using dimensional analysis.

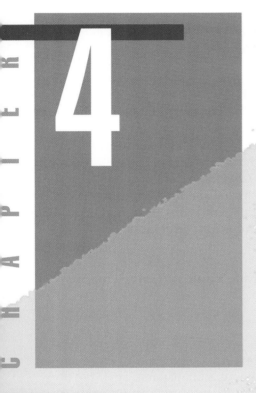

One-Factor
Medication Problems

Outline

INTERPRETATION OF MEDICATION ORDERS 60
Right Patient 60
Right Drug 60
Right Dosage 60
Right Route 61
Right Time 61
Exercise 4.1: Interpretation of Medication Orders 61
ONE-FACTOR MEDICATION PROBLEMS 62
Principles of Rounding 65
Exercise 4.2: One-Factor Medication Problems 68
COMPONENTS OF A DRUG LABEL 68
Identifying the Components 68
Exercise 4.3: Identifying the Components of Drug Labels 69
Solving Problems With Components of Drug Labels 71
Exercise 4.4: Problems with Components of Drug Labels 73
ADMINISTERING MEDICATION BY DIFFERENT ROUTES 74
Enteral Medications 74
Exercise 4.5: Administering Enteral Medications 79
Parenteral Medications 80
Exercise 4.6: Administering Parenteral Medications 85
Practice Problems for Chapter 4:
One-Factor Medication Problems 87
Post-Test for Chapter 4:
One-Factor Medication Problems 91
Answer Key for Chapter 4:
One-Factor Medication Problems 97

Objectives

After completing this chapter, you will be able to:

1. Interpret medication orders correctly, based on the five rights of medication administration.
2. Identify components from a drug label that are needed for accurate medication administration.
3. Describe the different routes of medication administration: tablets and capsules, liquids given by medicine cup or syringe, and parenteral injections using different types of syringes.
4. Calculate medication problems accurately from the one-factor–given quantity to the one-factor–wanted quantity using the sequential or random method of dimensional analysis.

PREVENTING MEDICATION ERRORS

Medication errors can be prevented by carefully adhering to these **five rights,** understanding the important concepts that apply to each right, and utilizing a nursing drug reference to provide accurate information for each medication administered.

Once you are able to interpret the important components of a medication order, you can perform accurate calculations for the correct dosage using dimensional analysis. If you cannot correctly interpret the components of a medication order (illegible prescription order), call the physician or nurse practitioner for clarification to prevent **medication errors.**

■ INTERPRETATION OF MEDICATION ORDERS

Physicians and nurse practitioners order medications using the **five rights** of medication administration including the:

1. Right **patient**
2. Right **drug**
3. Right **dosage**
4. Right **route**
5. Right **time**

Right Patient

Many medication errors can be prevented by correctly identifying the **right patient.** Patients in the hospital setting wear identification bands, whereas other facilities may use a photograph to identify the **right patient.**

Regardless of the identification method, the medication order must correspond to the identification of the patient. Checking identification and asking patients to state their names assists in reducing medication errors. It is also important to "listen" to the patient. If the patient states, "I don't take a blue pill," go back and check the medication order for correctness.

Right Drug

Medications can be ordered using their **trade name** or **generic name.**
Examples:

1. Tagamet® or cimetidine
2. Cipro® or ciprofloxacin hydrochloride

It is the responsibility of the nurse to look up a medication before administration to ensure that the **right drug** is being administered.

It is the responsibility of the nurse to know the classification of the drug being administered and that the drug corresponds with the patient diagnosis. Many drugs have similar names.
Example:

1. Celebrex® (an anti-inflammatory)
2. Celexa® (an antidepressant)

It is also the responsibility of the nurse to know the side effects of the drug being administered. The nurse must be aware of any patient allergies before medication administration to ensure safety of the patient. Allergies should be clearly recorded on medication records or a patient should wear an allergy bracelet.

Because it is impossible to know all medications, the nurse can use a nursing drug reference to look up medications to ensure accuracy and prevent medication errors.

Right Dosage

Medications are available in different dosages. It is the responsibility of the nurse to ensure that the **right dosage** is administered. The pharmacy may supply the exact dosage ordered or the dosage may need to be converted using a common equivalent or calculated based on the weight of the patient. If the medication must be reconstituted, the correct diluent must be used for reconstitution. If a patient is to receive a tablet but has difficulty swallowing, the nurse must obtain an order to have the medication changed to an elixir. Medication orders are to be administered exactly in the dosage ordered. A nursing drug reference assists with preventing medication errors by supplying information regarding the dosages of medications that can be safely administered to a patient based on age and weight.

Right Route

Medications may be administered by different routes including oral (tablets, capsules, or liquid), parenteral (intradermal, subcutaneous, intramuscular, or intravenous), or cutaneous (skin and mucous membranes). Improper medication administration techniques (crushing an enteric-coated tablet, opening a capsule, or giving an injection using the wrong route) are considered medication errors. A nursing drug reference provides information regarding the routes that can be safely used to administer medication and eliminate medication errors. It is the responsibility of the nurse to use this information to safely administer the medication to the patient using the **right route.**

Right Time

Medications are ordered and need to be administered at specific times to ensure the effective absorption of the medication. Failure to administer a medication on time or failure to document the administration of a medication is a medication error of omission. Some medications are ordered before meals (ac), after meals (pc), or at bedtime (hs). Other medications may be ordered based on frequency of time (once a day [qd], twice a day [bid], three times a day [tid], or four times a day [qid]). A nursing drug reference provides the nurse with the appropriate information to ensure that the medication is effectively and safely administered to eliminate a medication error based on adsorption. Most facilities allow a window of administration that is usually 30 minutes before or 30 minutes after the prescribed time. It is the responsibility of the nurse to use this information to safely administer the medication to the patient at the **right time.**

Once you are able to interpret the important components of an order for medication, you can perform accurate calculations for the correct drug dosage by using dimensional analysis.

Exercise 4.1	**Interpretation of Medication Orders**

(See page 97 for answers)

In the following medication orders, identify the five rights of medication administration.

1. Give gr 10 aspirin to Mrs. Clark orally every 4 hours as needed for fever.

   a. Right patient _____

   b. Right drug _____

   c. Right dosage _____

   d. Right route _____

   e. Right time _____

2. Administer PO to Mr. Smith, Advil (ibuprofen) 400 mg every 6 hours for arthritis.

   a. Right patient _____

   b. Right drug _____

PREVENTING MEDICATION ERRORS

Many believe that **documentation** should be the sixth "right of medication administration." Documentation is an important concept that can prevent medication errors related to over- or undermedication. The general rule of documentation is "if you didn't chart it . . . you didn't do it." Documentation should follow medication administration and include refusals, delays, and responses of medication administration.

(Exercise continues on page 62)

c. Right dosage   _____

d. Right route   _____

e. Right time   _____

3. Tylenol (acetaminophen) gr 10 PO every 4 hours for Mr. Jones prn for headache.

a. Right patient   _____

b. Right drug   _____

c. Right dosage   _____

d. Right route   _____

e. Right time   _____

■ ONE-FACTOR MEDICATION PROBLEMS

Medication problems can be easily solved using the five steps of dimensional analysis:

- The first step in interpreting any physician's order for medication is to identify the **given quantity** or the exact dosage that the physician ordered.
- The second step is to identify the **wanted quantity** or the answer to the medication problem.
- The third step is to establish the **unit path** from the given quantity to the wanted quantity, using equivalents as **conversion factors** to complete the problem. Identification of the available dosage of medicine (dose on hand) is considered part of the unit path.
- The fourth step is to set up the problem to cancel out unwanted units.
- The fifth step is to multiply the numerators, multiply the denominators, and divide the product of the numerators by the product of the denominators to provide the numerical value of the **wanted quantity** or answer to the problem.

You may choose to implement either the **sequential method** or the **random method** of dimensional analysis.

The **sequential method** requires that conversion factors be factored into the unit path in a logical, sequential method to cancel out a preceding unit.

The **random method** allows random placement of conversion factors within the unit path. The focus is on the correct placement of the conversion factor (dose on hand) in the unit path to correspond with the answer (wanted quantity). If the wanted quantity is tablets, then tablets must be in the numerator position in the unit path with the dosage in the denominator position.

Below is an example of a one-factor problem showing the placement of components used in dimensional analysis.

Unit Path

Given Quantity	Conversion Factor for Given Quantity	Conversion Computation	Wanted Quantity
10 gr	tablets	10	
	5 gr	5	= 2 tablets
	Conversion Factor for Wanted Quantity		

PREVENTING MEDICATION ERRORS

The **given quantity** is the **doctor's order** and should contain all **five rights** of the medication order.

EXAMPLE 4.1

The physician orders gr 10 aspirin orally every 4 hours, as needed for fever. The unit dose of medication on hand is gr 5 per tablet (5gr/tab).

▶ **How many tablets will you administer?**

Given quantity   = 10 gr
Wanted quantity = tablets
Dose on hand   = gr/tablet

STEP 1 Identify the *given quantity* (the physician's order).

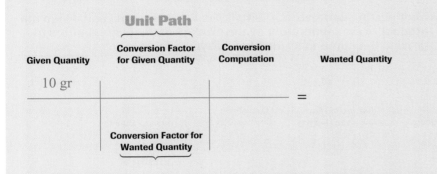

STEP 2 Identify the *wanted quantity* (the answer to the problem).

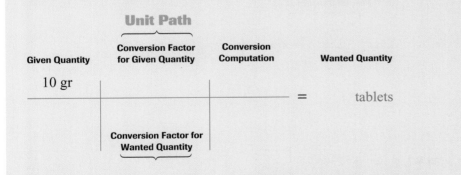

STEP 3 Establish the unit path from the given quantity to the wanted quantity using equivalents as conversion factors.

THINKING IT THROUGH

Both *10 gr* and *tablets* are numerators without a denominator. This is called a **one-factor** medication problem because the given quantity and the wanted quantity contain only numerators.

The dose on hand (5 gr/tablet) is an equivalent that is used as a conversion factor and is factored into the unit path.

The unwanted units (gr) can be canceled from the problem leaving the wanted quantity (tablets) in the numerator.

The **sequential method** of dimensional analysis has been used to factor in the dose on hand, which allows the previous unit (given quantity) to be canceled. When using the sequential method, the conversion factor that is factored in always cancels out the preceding unit.

(Example continues on page 64)

STEP 4 Set up the problem to allow cancellation of unwanted units and circle the wanted quantity within the unit path to demonstrate correct placement.

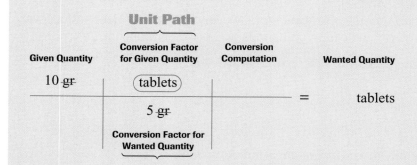

Unit Path

Given Quantity	Conversion Factor for Given Quantity	Conversion Computation	Wanted Quantity
10 gr	(tablets)		tablets
	5 gr		
	Conversion Factor for Wanted Quantity		

STEP 5 Multiply the numerators, multiply the denominators, and divide the product of the numerators by the product of the denominators to provide the numerical value for the wanted quantity.

Unit Path

Given Quantity	Conversion Factor for Given Quantity	Conversion Computation	Wanted Quantity
10 gr	(tablets)	10	2 tablets
	5 gr	5	
	Conversion Factor for Wanted Quantity		

▶▶▶ *2 tablets is the wanted quantity and the answer to the problem.*

PREVENTING MEDICATION ERRORS

When preparing to administer more than two tablets or capsules to a patient, always recalculate the answer to ensure the correct answer and prevent **medication errors.** Rarely does a patient receive more than two tablets or capsules of a medication. If more than two tablets or capsules are being administered, a different dosage of the medication should be discussed with the pharmacist.

THINKING IT THROUGH

The **sequential method** of dimensional analysis has been used to set up the problem. The unwanted units (mg) have been canceled from the unit path by correctly factoring in the dose on hand (200 mg/tablet). The same number of zeroes has also been canceled from the numerator and denominator.

EXAMPLE 4.2

Administer PO Advil (ibuprofen) 400 mg every 6 hours for arthritis. The dosage on hand is 200 mg/tablet.

▶ **How many tablets will you give?**

Given quantity   = 400 mg
Wanted quantity = tablets
Dose on hand   = 200 mg/tablet

STEP 1 Identify the *given quantity.*

400 mg	
	=

STEP 2 Identify the *wanted quantity.*

$$\frac{400 \text{ mg}}{\rule{2cm}{0pt}} \rule[0pt]{0pt}{1.5em} = \text{tablets}$$

STEP 3 Establish the unit path from the given quantity to the wanted quantity using equivalents as conversion factors.

$$\frac{400 \text{ mg}}{} \; \frac{\text{tablet}}{200 \text{ mg}} = \text{tablets}$$

STEP 4 Set up the problem to allow cancellation of unwanted units and circle the wanted quantity within the unit path to demonstrate correct placement.

$$\frac{400 \text{ m\!g}}{} \; \frac{\boxed{\text{tablet}}}{200 \text{ mg}} = \text{tablets}$$

STEP 5 Multiply the numerators, multiply the denominators, and divide the product of the numerators by the product of the denominators to provide the numerical value of the wanted quantity.

$$\frac{400 \text{ m\!g}}{} \; \frac{\boxed{\text{tablet}}}{200 \text{ m\!g}} \; \frac{4}{2} = 2 \text{ tablets}$$

▶ ▶ ▶ *2 tablets is the wanted quantity and the answer to the problem.*

Principles of Rounding

If an answer does not result in a whole number, but instead a decimal in the tenths (4.7) or hundredths (4.75), the answer must be rounded up or down to allow for administration of the medication.

If the tablets are scored, a half of the tablet can be administered. If a tablet is not scored, a decision must be made by the nurse whether to give one or two tablets. If a liquid medication to be administered involves decimals, then the nurse must make a decision regarding the amount of medication to be given.

If the number following the decimal is 5 or greater, then the number is rounded up.
Example in the tenths: 4.7 → 5
Example in the hundredths: 4.75 → 4.8

If the number following the decimal is less than 5, then the number is rounded down.
Example in the tenths: 4.4 → 4
Example in the hundredths: 4.42 → 4.4

PREVENTING MEDICATION ERRORS

Understanding the principles of rounding will prevent over- or undermedication, both of which are classified as **medication errors.**

EXAMPLE 4.3

Tylenol (acetaminophen) gr 10 PO every 4 hours for headache. The unit dose of medication on hand is 325 mg per caplet.

▶ **How many caplets will you give?**

Given quantity   = 10 gr
Wanted quantity = caplets
Dose on hand   = 325 mg/caplet

STEP 1 Identify the *given quantity.*

$$\dfrac{10\ gr}{} \qquad\qquad =$$

STEP 2 Identify the *wanted quantity.*

$$\dfrac{10\ gr}{} \qquad\qquad = caplets$$

STEP 3 Establish the *unit path* from the given quantity to the wanted quantity using equivalents as conversion factors.

$$\dfrac{10\ gr \quad\mid\quad 60\ mg \quad\mid\quad caplet}{\qquad\qquad 1\ gr \quad\mid\quad 325\ mg} = caplets$$

STEP 4 Set up the problem to allow cancellation of unwanted units and circle the wanted quantity within the unit path to demonstrate correct placement.

$$\dfrac{10\ \cancel{gr} \quad\mid\quad 60\ \cancel{mg} \quad\mid\quad \boxed{caplet}}{\qquad\qquad 1\ \cancel{gr} \quad\mid\quad 325\ \cancel{mg}} = caplets$$

STEP 5 Multiply the numerators, multiply the denominators, and divide the product of the numerators by the product of the denominators to provide the numerical value of the wanted quantity.

$$\dfrac{10\ \cancel{gr} \quad\mid\quad 60\ \cancel{mg} \quad\mid\quad \boxed{caplet} \quad\mid\quad 10\times 60 \quad\mid\quad 600}{\qquad\qquad 1\ \cancel{gr} \quad\mid\quad 325\ \cancel{mg} \quad\mid\quad 1\times 325 \quad\mid\quad 325} = 1.8\ caplets$$

▶▶▶   *1.8 caplets is the wanted quantity and the answer to the problem, but, by using the rounding rule, 2 caplets would be given.*

Dimensional analysis is a problem-solving method that uses critical think-ing, not a specific formula. Therefore, the important concept to remember is that *all* unwanted units must be canceled from the unit path. The **random method** of dimensional analysis can also be used when solving medication problems. When using the random method of dimensional analysis, the focus is on the correct placement of the conversion factor. It must correlate with the wanted quantity in the numerator portion of the unit path, without con-sidering the preceding units.

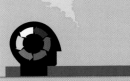

EXAMPLE 4.4
The random method of dimensional analysis will be used to calculate the answer for Example 4.3.

STEP 1 Identify the *given quantity.*

$$\frac{10 \text{ gr}}{} \Big| \qquad\qquad\qquad\qquad\qquad =$$

STEP 2 Identify the *wanted quantity.*

$$\frac{10 \text{ gr}}{} \Big| \qquad\qquad\qquad\qquad = \text{caplet}$$

STEP 3 Establish the *unit path* from the given quantity to the wanted quan-tity using equivalents as conversion factors.

$$\frac{10 \text{ gr}}{} \Bigg| \frac{\text{caplet}}{325 \text{ mg}} = \text{caplet}$$

STEP 4 Set up the problem to allow cancellation of unwanted units and cir-cle the wanted quantity within the unit path to demonstrate correct placement.

$$\frac{10 \text{ gr}}{} \Bigg| \frac{\boxed{\text{caplet}}}{325 \text{ mg}} \Bigg| \frac{60 \text{ mg}}{1 \text{ gr}} = \text{caplet}$$

STEP 5 Multiply the numerators, multiply the denominators, and divide the product of the numerators by the product of the denominators to provide the numerical value of the wanted quantity.

$$\frac{10 \text{ gr}}{} \Bigg| \frac{\boxed{\text{caplet}}}{325 \text{ mg}} \Bigg| \frac{60 \text{ mg}}{1 \text{ gr}} \Bigg| \frac{10 \times 60}{325 \times 1} \Bigg| \frac{600}{325} = 1.8 \text{ caplets}$$

▶ ▶ ▶   *1.8 caplets is the wanted quantity and the answer to the problem, but, by using the rounding rule, 2 caplets would be given.*

THINKING IT THROUGH

When using the random method, the focus is on the correct place-ment of the conversion factor to correspond with the wanted quantity. The problem is set up correctly as long as the dose on hand (caplet) correlates with the wanted quantity (caplet), both in the numerator.

   A conversion factor (1 gr = 60 mg) is factored into the problem to cancel out the unwanted units (gr and mg). The remaining unit (caplet) correlates with the wanted quantity.

Exercise 4.2   **One-Factor Medication Problems**
(See page 97 for answers)

1. The physician orders Achromycin (tetracycline) 0.25 g PO every 12 hours for acne. The dosage of medication on hand is 250 mg per capsule.

   ▶ **How many capsules will you give?** _____

2. Administer phenobarbital gr $\frac{1}{2}$ PO tid for sedation. The dosage on hand is 15 mg/tablet.

   ▶ **How many tablets will you give?** _____

3. Give 0.5 g Diuril PO bid for hypertension. Unit dose is 500 mg per tablet.

   ▶ **How many tablets will you give?** _____

4. Order: Restoril 0.03 g PO hs for sedation. Supply: Restoril 30-mg capsules.

   ▶ **How many capsules will you give?** _____

5. Order: Thorazine gr $\frac{1}{2}$ PO tid for singultus. Supply: Thorazine 30-mg capsules.

   ▶ **How many capsules will you give?** _____

PREVENTING MEDICATION ERRORS

Before administering any medication, the nurse should check the expiration date on the label. Administering a medication that has expired would be considered a **medication error.**

■ COMPONENTS OF A DRUG LABEL

All medications (stock and unit dose) are labeled with a drug label that includes specific information to assist in the accurate administration of the medication.

Identifying the Components

Information on the drug label includes:

- Name of the drug, including the trade name (name given by the pharmaceutical company identified with a trademark symbol) and the generic name (chemical name given to the drug)
- Dosage of medication (the amount of medication in each tablet, capsule, or liquid)
- Form of medication (tablet, capsule, or liquid)
- Expiration date (how long the medication will remain stable and safe to administer)
- Lot number or batch number (the manufacturer's batch series for this medication)
- Manufacturer (the pharmaceutical company that produced the medication)

EXAMPLE 4.5

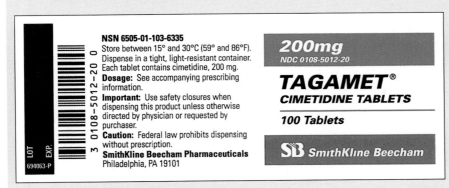

Courtesy of SmithKline Beecham Pharmaceuticals.

a. Trade name of the drug: Tagamet
b. Generic name of the drug: Cimetidine
c. Dosage of medication: 200 mg per tablet
d. Form of medication: 100 tablets
e. Expiration date:
f. Lot number or batch number:
g. Manufacturer: SmithKline Beecham Pharmaceuticals

Exercise 4.3   **Identifying the Components of Drug Labels**
(See pages 97–98 for answers)

1.

NDC 0026-8513-51
851310   4743   Printed in USA

CIPRO®

(ciprofloxacin hydrochloride)

Equivalent to
500 mg ciprofloxacin
100 Tablets

Caution: Federal (USA) law
prohibits dispensing without
a prescription.

Bayer
Bayer Corporation
Pharmaceutical Division
400 Morgan Lane
West Haven, CT 06516

Batch:
Expires:

DESCRIPTION: Each tablet contains ciprofloxacin
hydrochloride equivalent to 500 mg of ciprofloxacin.
DOSAGE: See accompanying literature for complete
information on dosage and administration.
RECOMMENDED STORAGE:
Store below 86°F (30°C).

PL500002   ©1995 Bayer Corporation
6505-01-333-4154
3   0026-8513-51   0

Courtesy of Bayer Corporation Pharmaceutical Division.

a. Trade name of the drug _____

b. Generic name of the drug _____

c. Dosage medication _____

(Exercise continues on page 70)

d. Form of medication _____

e. Expiration date _____

f. Batch number _____

g. Manufacturer _____

2.

Store at room temperature.
Container not for household use.
Dispense in a well-closed container.
Each capsule contains 100 mg
trimethobenzamide hydrochloride.
Dosage: See accompanying
prescribing information.
Important: Use safety closures
when dispensing this product
unless otherwise directed by
physician or requested by purchaser.
Manufactured by King
Pharmaceuticals, Inc., Bristol,
TN 37620 for **SmithKline Beecham
Pharmaceuticals**
Philadelphia, PA 19101

100mg
NDC 0029-4082-30

TIGAN®
TRIMETHO-
BENZAMIDE HCl

100 Capsules

SB SmithKline Beecham

Caution: Federal law prohibits
dispensing without prescription.

Courtesy of SmithKline Beecham Pharmaceuticals.

a. Trade name of the drug _____

b. Generic name of the drug _____

c. Dosage medication _____

d. Form of medication _____

e. Expiration date _____

f. Batch number _____

g. Manufacturer _____

3.

**Pharmacist: Dispense
in this container with
patient leaflet attached.**
See package insert
for complete product
information.
Keep container
tightly closed.
Store at controlled
room temperature
15° to 30° C
(59° to 86° F).
U.S. Patent No. 3,987,052
815 831 001

The Upjohn Co.
Kalamazoo, MI
49001, USA

Upjohn
NDC 0009-0010-37
10 Tablets

Halcion® C IV
Tablets
triazolam
tablets, USP

0.125mg

Caution: Federal law
prohibits dispensing
without prescription.

Courtesy of the Upjohn Company.

a. Trade name of the drug _____

b. Generic name of the drug _____

c. Dosage medication _____

d. Form of medication _____

e. Expiration date _____

f. Batch number _____

g. Manufacturer _____

Solving Problems With Components of Drug Labels

Once you are able to identify the components of a drug label, you can use critical thinking to solve problems with dimensional analysis.

The wanted quantity and the answer to the problem is 1.5 tablets. A scored tablet can be cut in half allowing the exact dosage to be administered. To prevent **medication errors,** always check with a pharmacist before altering the form of any medication.

EXAMPLE 4.6

The physician orders Cipro 750 mg PO every 12 hours for a bacterial infection.

▶ **How many tablets will you give?**

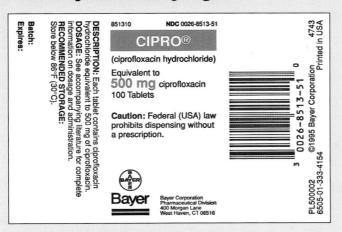

Courtesy of Bayer Corporation Pharmaceutical Division.

Given quantity   = 750 mg
Wanted quantity = tablets
Dose on hand   = 500 mg/tablet

Sequential method:

$$\frac{750 \text{ mg} \quad \boxed{\text{tablet}} \quad 75}{500 \text{ mg} \quad 50} = 1.5 \text{ tablets}$$

▶▶▶ *1.5 tablets is the wanted quantity and the answer to the problem.*

EXAMPLE 4.7

Administer Tigan 200 mg PO qid for nausea.

▶ **How many capsules will you give?**

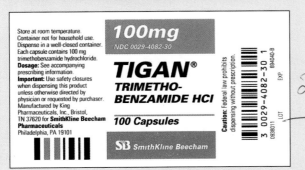

Courtesy of SmithKline Beecham Pharmaceuticals.

(Example continues on page 72)

Given quantity   = 200 mg
Wanted quantity = capsules
Dose on hand   = 100 mg/capsules

Sequential method:

$$\frac{200 \text{ mg}}{} \left| \frac{\text{capsules}}{100 \text{ mg}} \right| \frac{2}{1} = 2 \text{ capsules}$$

▶▶▶ *2 capsules is the wanted quantity and the answer to the problem.*

EXAMPLE 4.8

Order: Halcion 0.25 mg PO hs prn.

▶ **How many tablets will you give?**

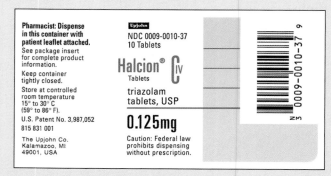

Pharmacist: Dispense
in this container with
patient leaflet attached.
See package insert
for complete product
information.
Keep container
tightly closed.
Store at controlled
room temperature
15° to 30° C
(59° to 86° F).
U.S. Patent No. 3,987,052
815 831 001
The Upjohn Co.
Kalamazoo, MI
49001, USA

Upjohn
NDC 0009-0010-37
10 Tablets

Halcion® C IV
Tablets
triazolam
tablets, USP

0.125mg

Caution: Federal law
prohibits dispensing
without prescription.

N3 0009-0010-37 9

Courtesy of the Upjohn Company.

Given quantity   = 0.25 mg
Wanted quantity = tablets
Dose on hand   = 0.125 mg/tablet

Sequential method:

$$\frac{0.25 \text{ mg}}{} \left| \frac{\text{tablet}}{0.125 \text{ mg}} \right| \frac{0.25}{0.125} = 2 \text{ tablets}$$

▶▶▶ *2 tablets is the wanted quantity and the answer to the problem.*

Exercise 4.4   **Problems With Components of Drug Labels**
(See page 98 for answers)

1. Order: methylphenidate 10 mg PO before breakfast and lunch for

attention-deficit hyperactivity disorder (ADHD)

▶ **How many tablets will you give?** _____

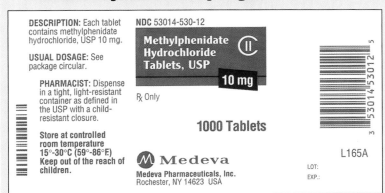

Courtesy of Medeva Pharmaceuticals.

2. Order: Xanax 500 mcg PO bid for anxiety

▶ **How many tablets will you give?** _____

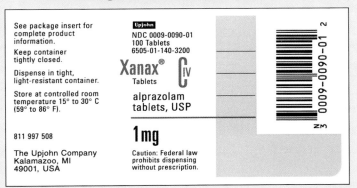

Courtesy of the Upjohn Company.

3. Order: Tolinase 375 mg PO every AM ac for type 2 diabetes mellitus

▶ **How many tablets will you give?** _____

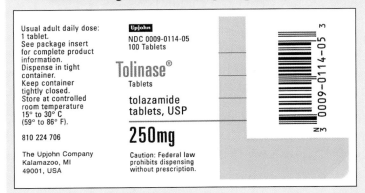

Courtesy of the Upjohn Company.

(Exercise continues on page 74)

4. Order: vitamin B₁₂ 2.5 mg daily as a daily vitamin supplement

▶ **How many tablets will you give?** _____

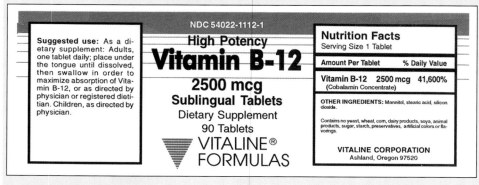

NDC 54022-1112-1

Suggested use: As a dietary supplement: Adults, one tablet daily; place under the tongue until dissolved, then swallow in order to maximize absorption of Vitamin B-12, or as directed by physician or registered dietitian. Children, as directed by physician.

High Potency
Vitamin B-12
2500 mcg
Sublingual Tablets
Dietary Supplement
90 Tablets
▼ **VITALINE®**
FORMULAS

Nutrition Facts
Serving Size 1 Tablet

Amount Per Tablet	% Daily Value
Vitamin B-12 2500 mcg 41,600% (Cobalamin Concentrate)	

OTHER INGREDIENTS: Mannitol, stearic acid, silicon dioxide.

Contains no yeast, wheat, corn, dairy products, soya, animal products, sugar, starch, preservatives, artificial colors or flavorings.

VITALINE CORPORATION
Ashland, Oregon 97520

Courtesy of Vitaline Corporation.

5. Order: Tigan 250 mg PO qid prn for nausea

▶ **How many capsules will you give?** _____

Store at room temperature. Container not for household use. Dispense in a well-closed container. Each capsule contains 250 mg trimethobenzamide hydrochloride.
Usual Adult Dosage: One capsule 3 or 4 times daily. See accompanying prescribing information.
Important: Use safety closures when dispensing this product unless otherwise directed by physician or requested by purchaser.
Manufactured by RSR Laboratories, Bristol, TN 37620 for
SmithKline Beecham Pharmaceuticals
Philadelphia, PA 19101

250mg
NDC 0029-4083-30

TIGAN®
TRIMETHO-BENZAMIDE HCl

100 Capsules

SB SmithKline Beecham

Caution: Federal law prohibits dispensing without prescription.

3 0029-4083-30 8
LOT   EXP

0938082
694077-A

Courtesy of SmithKline Beecham Pharmaceuticals.

■ ADMINISTERING MEDICATION BY DIFFERENT ROUTES

Medication may be administered by various routes, including oral, parenteral, or intravenous, involving tablets, capsules, or liquid.

Enteral Medications

Oral (PO) medications are administered using tablets, caplets, capsules, or liquid. Tablets and caplets may be scored, which permits a more accurate administration when one fourth or one half of a tablet must be given.

Tablets and caplets may also be enteric coated, which allows the medication to bypass disintegration in the stomach to decrease irritation, and then later break down in the small intestine for absorption. Enteric-coated tablets and caplets should never be crushed, because such medications irritate the stomach.

Capsules are usually of the time-release type, and these should never be crushed or opened because the medication would be immediately released into the system, instead of being released slowly over time.

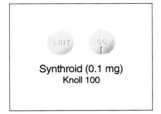

Synthroid (0.1 mg)
Knoll 100

Tablets: note scored tablet on right.

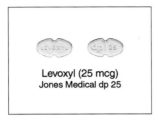

Levoxyl (25 mcg)
Jones Medical dp 25

Caplets: note scored caplet on right.

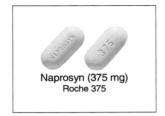

Naprosyn (375 mg)
Roche 375

Enteric-coated caplets.

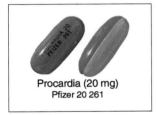

Procardia (20 mg)
Pfizer 20 261

Capsules.

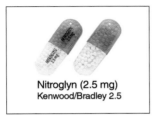

Nitroglyn (2.5 mg)
Kenwood/Bradley 2.5

Controlled-release capsules.

Liquid medication is accurately administered using a medication cup or medication syringe. The medication cup contains the common equivalents for the metric, apothecary, and household systems to permit adaptation of the medication's dosage for administration under various circumstances.

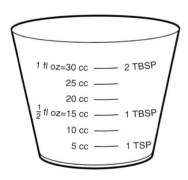

1 fl oz=30 cc —— 2 TBSP
25 cc ——
20 cc ——
½ fl oz=15 cc —— 1 TBSP
10 cc ——
5 cc —— 1 TSP

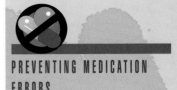

PREVENTING MEDICATION ERRORS

Opening capsules and adding the medication to applesauce or pudding would also be considered a **medication error** because the nurse did not administer the medication using the **right route.** The patient could receive an incorrect dosage of the medication as the medication quickly enters the gastrointestinal system.

EXAMPLE 4.9

Order: Tagamet 600 mg PO bid for gastrointestinal (GI) bleeding.

▶ **How many tsp will you give?**

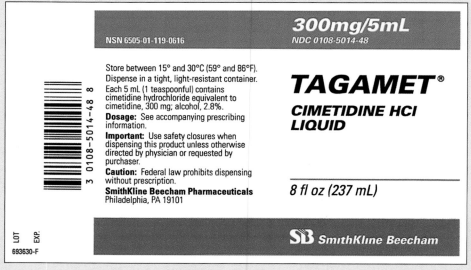

NSN 6505-01-119-0616

300mg/5mL

NDC 0108-5014-48

Store between 15° and 30°C (59° and 86°F).
Dispense in a tight, light-resistant container.
Each 5 mL (1 teaspoonful) contains
cimetidine hydrochloride equivalent to
cimetidine, 300 mg; alcohol, 2.8%.
Dosage: See accompanying prescribing
information.
Important: Use safety closures when
dispensing this product unless otherwise
directed by physician or requested by
purchaser.
Caution: Federal law prohibits dispensing
without prescription.
SmithKline Beecham Pharmaceuticals
Philadelphia, PA 19101

3 0108-5014-48 8

TAGAMET®

**CIMETIDINE HCl
LIQUID**

8 fl oz (237 mL)

SB SmithKline Beecham

LOT   EXP.
693630-F

Courtesy of SmithKline Beecham Pharmaceuticals.

Given quantity   = 600 mg
Wanted quantity = tsp
Dose on hand   = 300 mg/5 mL

Sequential method:

$$\frac{600 \text{ mg}}{} \left| \frac{5 \text{ mL}}{300 \text{ mg}} \right| \frac{\text{tsp}}{5 \text{ mL}} \left| \frac{6 \times 5}{3 \times 5} \right| \frac{30}{15} = 2 \text{ tsp}$$

▶▶▶ *2 tsp is the wanted quantity and the answer to the problem.*

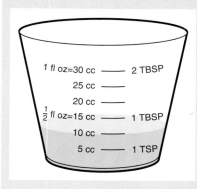

1 fl oz=30 cc ——— 2 TBSP
          25 cc ———
          20 cc ———
½ fl oz=15 cc ——— 1 TBSP
          10 cc ———
           5 cc ——— 1 TSP

EXAMPLE 4.10

Order: Compazine 10 mg PO qid for psychomotor agitation.

▶ **How many mL will you give?** _____

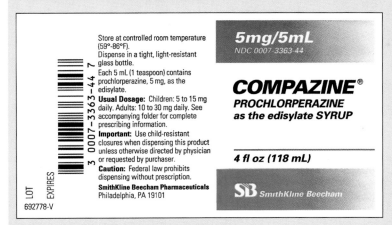

Courtesy of SmithKline Beecham Pharmaceuticals.

Given quantity   = 10 mg
Wanted quantity = mL
Dose on hand   = 5 mg/5 mL

Sequential method:

$$\frac{10\ \text{mg} \;\Big|\; 5\ \text{mL} \;\Big|\; 10}{\Big|\; 5\ \text{mg} \;\Big|} = 10\ \text{mL}$$

▶▶▶   *10 mL is the wanted quantity and the answer to the problem.*

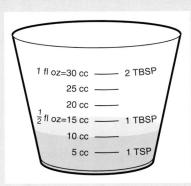

EXAMPLE 4.11

Order: Tegretol 100 mg PO qid for convulsions.

▶ **How many tsp will you give?** _____

NDC 58887-019-76   FSC 1841
6505-01-302-4467

Tegretol®
carbamazepine USP
Suspension
100 mg/5 ml

3 58887-019-76 0

EXP
LOT

450 ml

**Dispense in tight, light-resistant
container (USP).**

Caution: Federal law prohibits
dispensing without prescription.

BASEL
Pharmaceuticals

Each 5 ml contains 100 mg carbamazepine USP.
Shake well before using.
Dosage: See package insert.
Do not store above 86°F (30°C).

BASEL Pharmaceuticals
Division of CIBA-GEIGY Corporation
Summit, New Jersey 07901

643754

Courtesy of Basel Pharmaceuticals.

Given quantity   = 100 mg
Wanted quantity = tsp
Dose on hand   = 100 mg/5 mL

Random method:

$$\frac{100 \text{ mg}}{} \; \left| \; \frac{1 \text{ tsp}}{5 \text{ mL}} \; \right| \; \frac{5 \text{ mL}}{100 \text{ mg}} \; \left| \; \frac{1}{} \right. = 1 \text{ tsp}$$

▶▶▶ *1 tsp is the wanted quantity and the answer to the problem.*

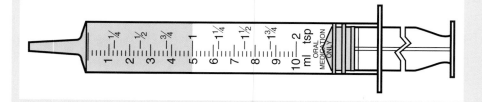

Exercise 4.5 **Administering Enteral Medications**
(See pages 98–99 for answers)

1. Order: phenobarbital gr $\frac{1}{2}$ PO daily for convulsions

   On hand: 20 mg/5 mL

   ▶ **How many mL will you give?** _____

   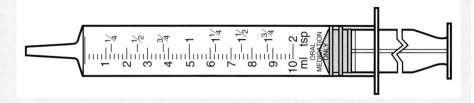

2. Order: Zantac 0.15 g PO bid for ulcers

   On hand: 15 mg/mL

   ▶ **How many tsp will you give?** _____

   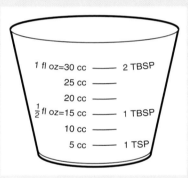

3. Order: Dilaudid 3 mg PO every 3 hours prn for pain

   On hand: Dilaudid Liquid 1 mg/mL

   ▶ **How many mL will you give?** _____

   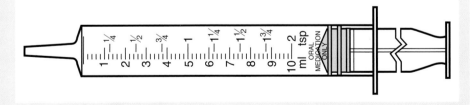

(Exercise continues on page 80)

4. Order: lactulose 20 g PO tid for hepatic encephalopathy

On hand: lactulose 10 g/15 mL

▶ **How many oz will you give?** _____

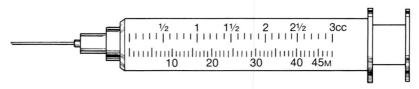

Parenteral Medications

Medications may also be ordered by the physician for the parenteral route of administration, including subcutaneous (SQ), intramuscular (IM), and intravenous (IV). Parenteral medications are sterile solutions obtained from vials or ampules and are administered using a syringe or prefilled syringes. The three syringes most often used are:

1. 3-cc syringe (used for a variety of medications requiring administration of doses from 0.2 to 3 cc).

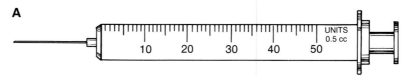

3-cc syringe

2. Insulin syringe (used specifically to administer insulin). Two types are illustrated below **A.** 0.5-mL (cc) low-dose syringe for U-100 insulin and **B.** 1-mL (cc) syringe for U-100 insulin.

A

0.5-mL (cc) low-dose syringe

B

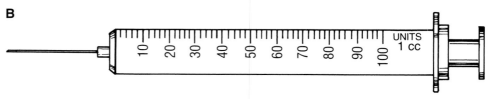

1-mL (cc) syringe

3. Tuberculin syringe (used for a variety of medications requiring administration of doses from 0.1 to 1 cc). Marked in hundredths to allow for
rounding or exact dosage (eg, 0.75 mL).

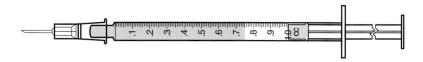

Tuberculin syringe

EXAMPLE 4.12
Order: Tigan 100 mg IM qid for nausea.

▶ **How many mL will you give?** _____

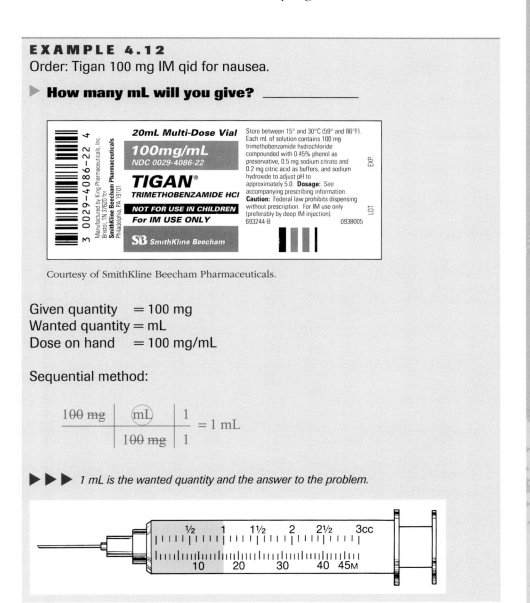

Courtesy of SmithKline Beecham Pharmaceuticals.

Given quantity   = 100 mg
Wanted quantity = mL
Dose on hand   = 100 mg/mL

Sequential method:

$$\frac{100 \text{ mg}}{1} \times \frac{\text{mL}}{100 \text{ mg}} \times \frac{1}{1} = 1 \text{ mL}$$

▶▶▶ *1 mL is the wanted quantity and the answer to the problem.*

EXAMPLE 4.13

Order: Compazine 10 mg IM every 4 hours for psychoses.

▶ **How many mL will you give?** _____

Store below 86°F. Do not freeze.
Protect from light. Discard if markedly discolored.
Each mL contains, in aqueous solution, prochlorper-
azine, 5 mg, as the edisylate; sodium biphosphate,
5 mg; sodium tartrate, 12 mg; sodium saccharin,
0.9 mg; benzyl alcohol, 0.75%, as preservative.
Dosage: For deep I.M. or I.V. injection.
See accompanying prescribing information.
Caution: Federal law prohibits dispensing without
prescription.
SmithKline Beecham Pharmaceuticals
693793-AD   Philadelphia, PA 19101

LOT
EXP:

10mL Multi-Dose Vial
5mg/mL
NDC 0007-3343-01
COMPAZINE®
PROCHLORPERAZINE
as the edisylate INJECTION

SB SmithKline Beecham

Courtesy of SmithKline Beecham Pharmaceuticals.

Given quantity   = 10 mg
Wanted quantity = mL
Dose on hand   = 5 mg/mL

Sequential method:

$$\frac{10 \text{ mg}}{} \left| \frac{\text{mL}}{5 \text{ mg}} \right| \frac{10}{5} = 2 \text{ mL}$$

▶▶▶ *2 mL is the wanted quantity and the answer to the problem.*

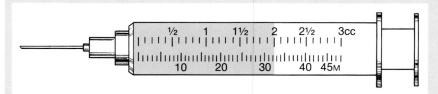

EXAMPLE 4.14

Order: morphine sulfate, $\frac{1}{4}$ gr every 4 hours prn for pain.

▶ **How many mL will you give?** _____

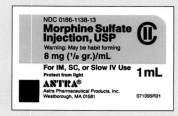

NDC 0186-1138-13
Morphine Sulfate
Injection, USP Ⓒ
Warning: May be habit forming
8 mg (¹/₈ gr.)/mL
For IM, SC, or Slow IV Use
Protect from light   **1mL**
ANTRA®
Astra Pharmaceutical Products, Inc.
Westborough, MA 01581   071095R01

Courtesy of Astra Pharmaceutical Products.

Given quantity $= \frac{1}{4}$ gr
Wanted quantity $=$ mL
Dose on hand $= 8$ mg/mL or $\frac{1}{8}$ gr/mL

Random method:

$$\frac{\frac{1}{4} \text{ gr}}{} \left| \frac{\text{mL}}{8 \text{ mg}} \right| \frac{60 \text{ mg}}{1 \text{ gr}} \left| \frac{\frac{1}{4} \times \frac{60}{1}}{8 \times 1} \right| \frac{\frac{60}{4}}{8} \left| \frac{15}{8} \right. = 1.87 \text{ mL or } 1.9 \text{ mL}$$

▶▶▶ *1.87 mL is the wanted quantity and the answer to the problem, but, by using the rounding rule, 1.9 mL would be given.*

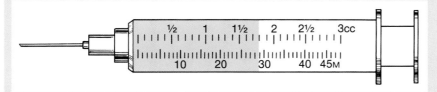

EXAMPLE 4.15

Order: NPH human insulin 20 units SQ every AM for type 1 diabetes mellitus.

▶ **How many units will you give?** _____

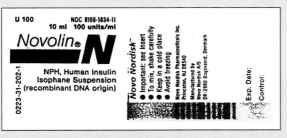

Courtesy of Novo Nordisk Pharmaceutical.

Sequential method:

$$\frac{20 \text{ units}}{} = 20 \text{ units}$$

▶▶▶ *20 units is the wanted quantity and the answer to the problem.*

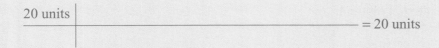

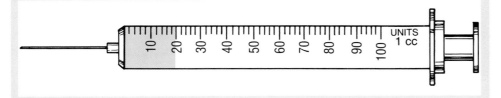

Heparin is an anticoagulant that is used to decrease the clotting ability of the blood and help prevent harmful clots from forming in the blood vessels. Although heparin is commonly referred to as a blood thinner, it does not dissolve blood clots that have already formed. Heparin may help prevent blood clots from becoming larger and causing more serious problems to the heart or lungs.

Heparin is administered using a tuberculin syringe, which is calibrated from 0.1 to 1 cc. This allows for more accurate administration of medication dosages of less than 1 cc.

EXAMPLE 4.16

Order: NPH human insulin 45 units SQ every AM for type 1 diabetes mellitus.

▶ **How many units will you give?** _____

U 100   NDC 0169-1834-11
10 ml   100 units/ml

Novolin® N

NPH, Human Insulin
Isophane Suspension
(recombinant DNA origin)

0223-31-202-1

Novo Nordisk™
● Important: see insert
● To mix, shake carefully
● Keep in a cold place
● Avoid freezing

Novo Nordisk Pharmaceuticals Inc.
Princeton, NJ 08540
Manufactured by
Novo Nordisk A/S
DK-2880 Bagsvaerd, Denmark

Exp. Date:
Control:

Courtesy of Novo Nordisk Pharmaceutical.

Sequential method:

45 units |―――――――――――――――――――――――――― = 45 units

UNITS
0.5 cc

10   20   30   40   50

It is also the responsibility of the nurse to be familiar with the different types of anticoagulants (heparin, Warfarin, and Coumadin) to ensure patient safety and prevent **medication errors.** The nurse needs to know which laboratory value to monitor (PT, PTT, INR) and which antidote (protamine sulfate or vitamin K) to have available for emergencies.

EXAMPLE 4.17

Order: heparin 5000 units SQ bid for prevention of thrombi. On hand: heparin 10,000 units/mL.

▶ **How many mL will you give?** _____

Sequential method:

$$\frac{5000 \text{ units}}{} \;\Big|\; \frac{mL}{10{,}000 \text{ units}} \;\Big|\; \frac{5}{10} = 0.5 \text{ mL}$$

▶▶▶ *0.5 mL is the wanted quantity and the answer to the problem.*

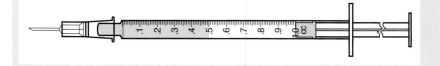

Exercise 4.6   **Administering Parenteral Medications**
(See page 99 for answers)

1. Order: atropine sulfate 300 mcg IM for preoperative medication.

▶ **How many mL will you give?** _____

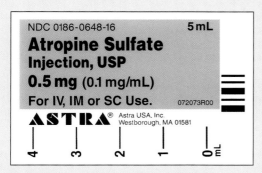

NDC 0186-0648-16   **5 mL**

Atropine Sulfate
Injection, USP
0.5 mg (0.1 mg/mL)
For IV, IM or SC Use.   072073R00

ASTRA® Astra USA, Inc.
Westborough, MA 01581

Courtesy of Astra Pharmaceutical Products.

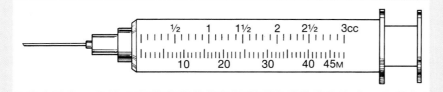

2. Order: hydromorphone 3 mg IM every 4 hours for pain.

▶ **How many mL will you give?** _____

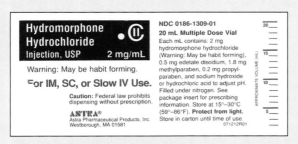

**Hydromorphone
Hydrochloride**
Injection, USP   **2 mg/mL**

Warning: May be habit forming.

For IM, SC, or Slow IV Use.

Caution: Federal law prohibits
dispensing without prescription.
ASTRA®
Astra Pharmaceutical Products, Inc.
Westborough, MA 01581

NDC 0186-1309-01
20 mL Multiple Dose Vial
Each mL contains: 2 mg
hydromorphone hydrochloride
(Warning: May be habit forming),
0.5 mg edetate disodium, 1.8 mg
methylparaben, 0.2 mg propyl-
paraben, and sodium hydroxide
or hydrochloric acid to adjust pH.
Filled under nitrogen. See
package insert for prescribing
information. Store at 15°–30°C
(59°–86°F). **Protect from light.**
Store in carton until time of use.
071212R01

Courtesy of Astra Pharmaceutical Products.

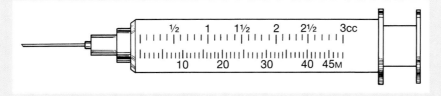

(Exercise continues on page 86)

3. Order: meperidine 35 mg IV every hour for pain.

▶ **How many mL will you give?** _____

NDC 0338-2691-75

Meperidine HCl Injection, USP

Warning – May be habit forming.

C II

50 mL

6468020
Reorder Number

Baxter

500 mg (10 mg/mL)

FOR INTRAVENOUS USE
USUAL DOSAGE: SEE PACKAGE INSERT FOR DOSAGE INFORMATION
SINGLE USE/NO BACTERIOSTAT OR ANTIMICROBIAL AGENTS ADDED

Each mL contains: 10 mg meperidine HCl with sodium hydroxide and/or hydrochloric acid to adjust pH 3.5–6.0.

Caution: Federal law (U.S.A.) prohibits dispensing without prescription.
For use with PCA syringe pumps manufactured by Baxter Healthcare Corporation.
Distributed by: Baxter Healthcare Corporation, Deerfield, IL 60015
Manufactured by: Astra USA, Inc., Westborough, MA 01581

071434R03

Patient/I.D. #

GRADUATIONS ARE APPROXIMATE

500 450 400 350 300 250 200 150 100 50 mg
50 45 40 35 30 25 20 15 10 5 mL

Courtesy of Baxter Pharmaceuticals.

4. Order: regular insulin 10 units SQ every AM for type 1 diabetes mellitus.

On hand: regular insulin 100 units/mL.

▶ **How many units will you give?** _____

5. Order: heparin 8000 units SQ bid for prevention of thrombi.

On hand: heparin 10,000 units/mL.

▶ **How many mL will you give?** _____

S U M M A R Y

This chapter has taught you to interpret medication orders and drug labels and to calculate one-factor medication problems using dimensional analysis. To demonstrate your ability to interpret correctly and calculate accurately, complete the following practice problems.

| **Practice Problems for Chapter 4** | **One-Factor Medication Problems** |

(See pages 99–100 for answers)

1. The physician orders Tigan 0.2 g IM qid for nausea. The dosage of medication on hand is a multiple-dose vial labeled 100 mg/mL.

   ▶ **How many mL will you give?** _____

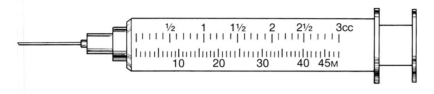

2. A physician orders Thorazine 50 mg tid prn for singultus. The dose on hand is Thorazine 25-mg tablets.

   ▶ **How many tablets will you give?** _____

3. Order: Orinase 1 g PO bid for type 2 diabetes mellitus

   ▶ **How many tablets will you give?** _____

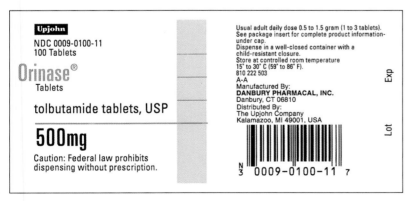

Courtesy of the Upjohn Company.

4. Order: Persantine 50 mg PO qid for prevention of thromboembolism

▶ **How many tablets will you give?** _____

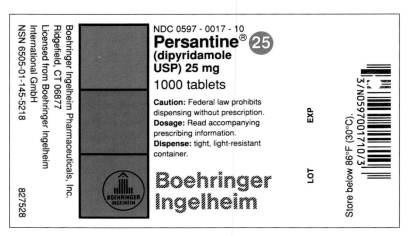

NDC 0597 - 0017 - 10
Persantine® 25
(dipyridamole
USP) 25 mg
1000 tablets

Caution: Federal law prohibits dispensing without prescription.
Dosage: Read accompanying prescribing information.
Dispense: tight, light-resistant container.

EXP

LOT

Store below 86°F (30°C).

Boehringer Ingelheim

Boehringer Ingelheim Pharmaceuticals, Inc.
Ridgefield, CT 06877
Licensed from Boehringer Ingelheim International GmbH
NSN 6505-01-145-5218

827528

Courtesy of Boehringer Ingelheim Pharmaceuticals.

5. Order: NPH insulin 56 units SQ every AM for type 1 diabetes mellitus

On hand: NPH insulin 100 units/mL

▶ **How many units will you give?** _____

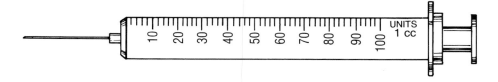

6. Order: heparin 7500 units SQ bid for prevention of thrombi

On hand: heparin 10,000 units/mL

▶ **How many mL will you give?** _____

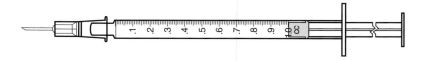

7. Order: Augmentin 500 mg PO every 8 hours for infection.

▶ **How many mL will you give?** _____

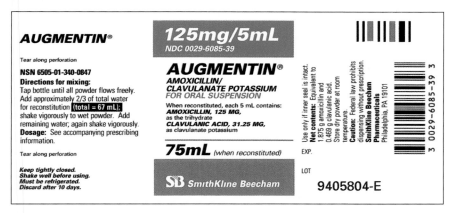

Courtesy of SmithKline Beecham Pharmaceuticals.

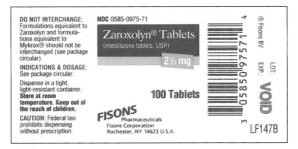

8. Order: Zaroxolyn 5 mg PO every AM for hypertension

▶ **How many tablets will you give?** _____

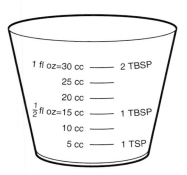

Courtesy of Fisons Pharmaceuticals.

9. Order: methylphenidate (Ritalin) 10 mg PO tid for attention-deficit hyperactivity disorder (ADHD)

▶ **How many tablets will you give?** _____

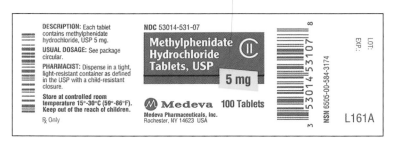

Courtesy of Medeva Pharmaceuticals.

10. Order: meperidine 50 mg IM every 3 hours prn for pain.

On hand: meperidine 100 mg/mL

▶ **How many mL will you give?** _____

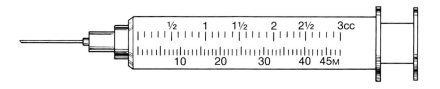

Chapter 4 Post-Test: One-Factor Medication Problems

Name _____ **Date** _____

1. Order: Micronase 1.25 mg PO daily for non-insulin-dependent diabetes mellitus

   ▶ **How many tablets will you give?** _____

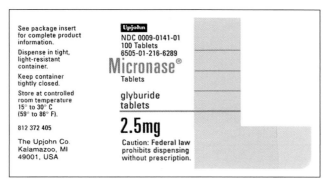

Courtesy of the Upjohn Company.

2. Order: Tegretol 50 mg PO qid for seizures

   ▶ **How many tablets will you give?** _____

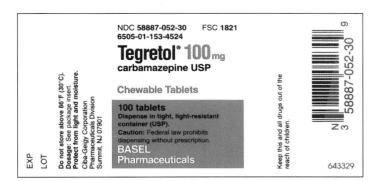

Courtesy of Basel Pharmaceuticals.

3. Order: acetaminophen 240 mg PO every 4 hours prn for moderate pain

▶ **How many milliliters will you give?** _____

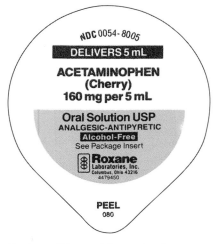

Courtesy of Roxane Laboratories, Inc.

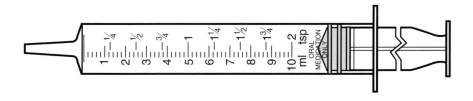

4. Order: lactulose 30 g PO qid for hepatic encephalopathy

▶ **How many milliliters will you give?** _____

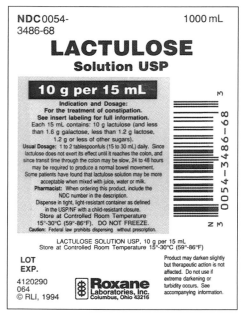
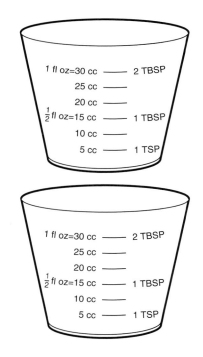

Courtesy of Roxane Laboratories, Inc.

5. Order: Tagamet 300 mg PO qid for short-term treatment of active ulcers

▶ **How many teaspoons will you give?**

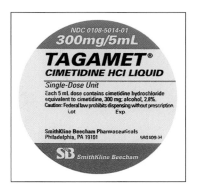

Courtesy of SmithKline Beecham
Pharmaceuticals.

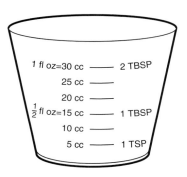

6. Order: Tigan 0.2 g IM tid prn for nausea

▶ **How many milliliters will you give?**

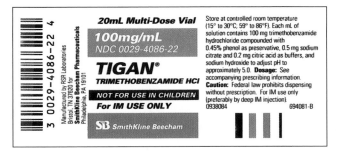

Courtesy of SmithKline Beecham Pharmaceuticals.

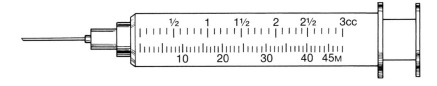

7. Order: hydromorphone 3 mg IM every 3 hours for pain

▶ **How many milliliters will you give?** _____

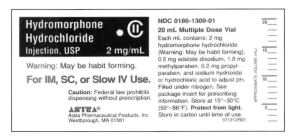

Courtesy of Astra Pharmaceutical Products.

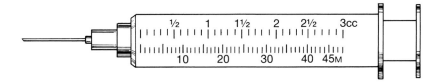

8. Order: magnesium sulfate 1000 mg IM in each buttock for

hypomagnesemia

▶ **How many milliliters will you give?** _____

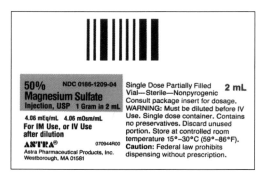

Courtesy of Astra Pharmaceutical Products.

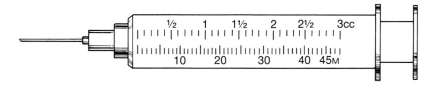

9. Order: naloxone HCl 200 mcg IV stat for respiratory depression

▶ **How many milliliters will you give?**

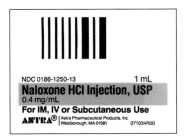

Courtesy of Astra Pharmaceutical
Products.

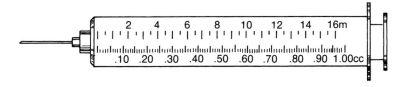

10. Order: Solu-Medrol 40 mg IM daily for autoimmune disorder

▶ **How many milliliters will you give?**

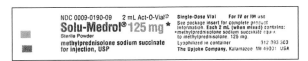

Courtesy of the Upjohn Company.

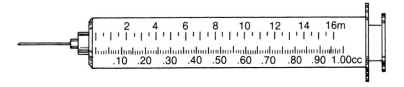

ANSWER KEY FOR CHAPTER 4: ONE-FACTOR MEDICATION PROBLEMS

Exercise 4.1 Interpretation of Medication Orders

1

a. Right patient   Mrs. C. Clark
b. Right drug   Aspirin for fever
c. Right dosage   gr 10
d. Right route   orally (PO)
e. Right time   every 4 hr as needed (prn)

2

a. Right patient   Mr. S. Smith
b. Right drug   Advil (ibuprofen) for arthritis
c. Right dosage   400 mg
d. Right route   PO (orally)
e. Right time   every 6 hr

3

a. Right patient   Mr. J. Jones
b. Right drug   Tylenol (acetaminophen) for headache
c. Right dosage   gr 10
d. Right route   PO (orally)
e. Right time   every 4 hr prn

Exercise 4.2 One-Factor Medication Problems

1. Sequential method:

$$\frac{0.25\ \text{g}}{} \left|\frac{1000\ \text{mg}}{1\ \text{g}}\right| \frac{\text{capsule}}{250\ \text{mg}} \left|\frac{0.25 \times 100}{1 \times 25}\right| \frac{25}{25} = 1\ \text{capsule}$$

Random method:

$$\frac{0.25\ \text{g}}{} \left|\frac{\text{capsule}}{250\ \text{mg}}\right| \frac{1000\ \text{mg}}{1\ \text{g}} \left|\frac{0.25 \times 100}{25 \times 1}\right| \frac{25}{25} = 1\ \text{capsule}$$

2. Sequential method:

$$\frac{\frac{1}{2}\ \text{gr}}{} \left|\frac{60\ \text{mg}}{1\ \text{gr}}\right| \frac{\text{tablet}}{15\ \text{mg}} \left|\frac{\frac{1}{2} \times \frac{60}{1}}{1 \times 15}\right| \frac{\frac{60}{2}}{15} \frac{30}{15} = 2\ \text{tablets}$$

Random method:

$$\frac{\frac{1}{2}\ \text{gr}}{} \left|\frac{\text{tablet}}{15\ \text{mg}}\right| \frac{60\ \text{mg}}{1\ \text{gr}} \left|\frac{\frac{1}{2} \times \frac{60}{1}}{15 \times 1}\right| \frac{\frac{60}{2}}{15} \frac{30}{15} = 2\ \text{tablets}$$

3. Sequential method:

$$\frac{0.5\ \text{g}}{} \left|\frac{1000\ \text{mg}}{1\ \text{g}}\right| \frac{\text{tablet}}{500\ \text{mg}} \left|\frac{0.5 \times 10}{1 \times 5}\right| \frac{5}{5} = 1\ \text{tablet}$$

Random method:

$$\frac{0.5\ \text{g}}{} \left|\frac{\text{tablet}}{500\ \text{mg}}\right| \frac{1000\ \text{mg}}{1\ \text{g}} \left|\frac{0.5 \times 10}{5 \times 1}\right| \frac{5}{5} = 1\ \text{tablet}$$

4. Sequential method:

$$\frac{0.03\ \text{g}}{} \left|\frac{1000\ \text{mg}}{1\ \text{g}}\right| \frac{\text{capsules}}{30\ \text{mg}} \left|\frac{0.03 \times 100}{1 \times 3}\right| \frac{3}{3} = 1\ \text{capsule}$$

Random method:

$$\frac{0.03\ \text{g}}{} \left|\frac{\text{capsules}}{30\ \text{mg}}\right| \frac{1000\ \text{mg}}{1\ \text{g}} \left|\frac{0.03 \times 100}{3 \times 1}\right| \frac{3}{3} = 1\ \text{capsule}$$

5. Sequential method:

$$\frac{\frac{1}{2}\ \text{gr}}{} \left|\frac{60\ \text{mg}}{1\ \text{gr}}\right| \frac{\text{capsules}}{30\ \text{mg}} \left|\frac{\frac{1}{2} \times \frac{60}{1}}{1 \times 30}\right| \frac{\frac{60}{2}}{30} \frac{30}{30} = 1\ \text{capsule}$$

Random method:

$$\frac{\frac{1}{2}\ \text{gr}}{} \left|\frac{\text{capsules}}{30\ \text{mg}}\right| \frac{60\ \text{mg}}{1\ \text{gr}} \left|\frac{\frac{1}{2} \times \frac{60}{1}}{30 \times 1}\right| \frac{\frac{60}{2}}{30} \frac{30}{30} = 1\ \text{capsule}$$

Exercise 4.3 Identifying the Components of Drug Labels

1

a. Cipro
b. Ciprofloxacin hydrochloride
c. 500 mg per tablet
d. 100 tablets
e. *Not listed on the label
f. *Not listed on the label
g. Bayer Corporation, Pharmaceutical Division

2
a. Tigan
b. Trimethobenzamide hydrochloride
c. 100 mg per capsule
d. 100 capsules
e. *Not listed on the label
f. *Not listed on the label
g. SmithKline Beecham Pharmaceuticals

3
a. Halcion
b. Triazolam
c. 0.125 mg per tablet
d. 10 tablets
e. *Not listed on the label
f. *Not listed on the label
g. The Upjohn Company

Exercise 4.4 Problems With Components of Drug Labels

1. Sequential method:

$$\frac{10 \text{ mg}}{} \left| \frac{\text{tablet}}{10 \text{ mg}} \right| \frac{10}{10} = 1 \text{ tablet}$$

2. Random method:

$$\frac{500 \text{ mcg}}{} \left| \frac{\text{tablet}}{1 \text{ mg}} \right| \frac{1 \text{ mg}}{1000 \text{ mcg}} \left| \frac{5}{10} \right. = \frac{1}{2} \text{ tablet}$$

3. Sequential method:

$$\frac{375 \text{ mg}}{} \left| \frac{\text{tablet}}{250 \text{ mg}} \right| \frac{375}{250} = 1\frac{1}{2} \text{ tablets}$$

4. Random method:

$$\frac{2.5 \text{ mg}}{} \left| \frac{\text{tablet}}{2500 \text{ mcg}} \right| \frac{1000 \text{ mcg}}{1 \text{ mg}} \left| \frac{2.5 \times 10}{25 \times 1} \right| \frac{25}{25} = 1 \text{ tablet}$$

5. Sequential method:

$$\frac{250 \text{ mg}}{} \left| \frac{\text{capsule}}{250 \text{ mg}} \right| \frac{25}{25} = 1 \text{ capsule}$$

Exercise 4.5 Administering Enteral Medications

1. Random method:

$$\frac{\frac{1}{2} \text{ gr}}{} \left| \frac{5 \text{ mL}}{20 \text{ mg}} \right| \frac{60 \text{ mg}}{1 \text{ gr}} \left| \frac{\frac{1}{2} \times \frac{5}{1} \times \frac{6}{1}}{2 \times 1} \right| \frac{30}{2} \left| \frac{15}{2} \right. = 7.5 \text{ mL}$$

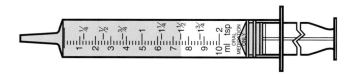

2. Sequential method:

$$\frac{0.15 \text{ g}}{} \left| \frac{1000 \text{ mg}}{1 \text{ g}} \right| \frac{\text{mL}}{15 \text{ mg}} \left| \frac{1 \text{ tsp}}{5 \text{ mL}} \right| \frac{0.15 \times 1000}{15 \times 5} \left| \frac{150}{75} \right. = 2 \text{ tsp}$$

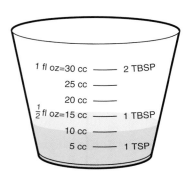

3. Sequential method:

$$\frac{3 \text{ mg}}{} \left| \frac{\text{mL}}{1 \text{ mg}} \right| \frac{3}{1} = 3 \text{ mL}$$

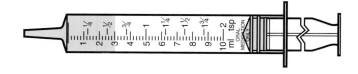

4. Sequential method:

$$\frac{20 \text{ g}}{} \bigg| \frac{15 \text{ mL}}{10 \text{ g}} \bigg| \frac{1 \text{ oz}}{30 \text{ mL}} \bigg| \frac{2 \times 15 \times 1}{1 \times 30} \bigg| \frac{30}{30} = 1 \text{ oz}$$

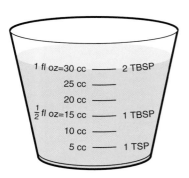

Exercise 4.6 Administering Parenteral Medications

1. Random method

$$\frac{300 \text{ mcg}}{} \bigg| \frac{\text{mL}}{0.1 \text{ mg}} \bigg| \frac{1 \text{ mg}}{1000 \text{ mcg}} \bigg| \frac{3 \times 1}{0.1 \times 10} \bigg| \frac{3}{1} = 3 \text{ mL}$$

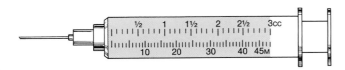

2. Sequential method:

$$\frac{3 \text{ mg}}{} \bigg| \frac{\text{mL}}{2 \text{ mg}} \bigg| \frac{3}{2} = 1.5 \text{ mL}$$

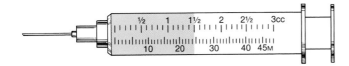

3. Sequential method:

$$\frac{35 \text{ mg}}{} \bigg| \frac{\text{mL}}{10 \text{ mg}} \bigg| \frac{35}{10} = 3.5 \text{ mL}$$

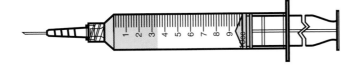

4. Sequential method:

$$\frac{10 \text{ units}}{} \bigg|\qquad\qquad = 10 \text{ units}$$

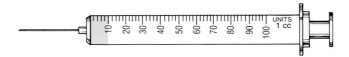

5. Sequential method:

$$\frac{8000 \text{ units}}{} \bigg| \frac{\text{mL}}{10,000 \text{ units}} \bigg| \frac{8}{10} = 0.8 \text{ mL}$$

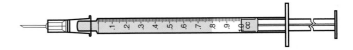

Practice Problems

1. Random method:

$$\frac{0.2 \text{ g}}{} \bigg| \frac{\text{mL}}{100 \text{ mg}} \bigg| \frac{1000 \text{ mg}}{1 \text{ g}} \bigg| \frac{0.2 \times 10}{1 \times 1} \bigg| \frac{2}{1} = 2 \text{ mL}$$

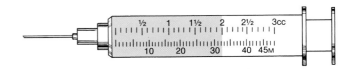

2. Sequential method:

$$\frac{50 \text{ mg}}{} \bigg| \frac{\text{tablet}}{25 \text{ mg}} \bigg| \frac{50}{25} = 2 \text{ tablets}$$

3. Random method:

$$\frac{1 \text{ g}}{} \bigg| \frac{\text{tablet}}{500 \text{ mg}} \bigg| \frac{1000 \text{ mg}}{1 \text{ g}} \bigg| \frac{1 \times 10}{5 \times 1} \bigg| \frac{10}{5} = 2 \text{ tablets}$$

4. Random method:

$$\frac{50 \text{ mg}}{} \bigg| \frac{\text{tablet}}{25 \text{ mg}} \bigg| \frac{50}{25} = 2 \text{ tablets}$$

5. Sequential method:

$$\frac{56 \text{ units}}{} = 56 \text{ units}$$

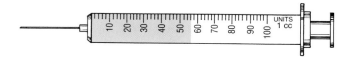

6. Sequential method:

$$\frac{7500 \text{ units}}{} \left| \frac{\text{mL}}{10000 \text{ units}} \right| \frac{75}{100} = 0.75 \text{ mL}$$

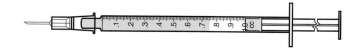

7. Sequential method:

$$\frac{500 \text{ mg}}{} \left| \frac{5 \text{ mL}}{125 \text{ mg}} \right| \frac{500 \times 5}{125} \left| \frac{2500}{125} \right. = 20 \text{ mL}$$

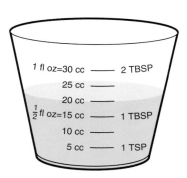

8. Sequential method:

$$\frac{5 \text{ mg}}{} \left| \frac{\text{tablet}}{2.5 \text{ mg}} \right| \frac{5}{2.5} = 2 \text{ tablets}$$

9. Sequential method:

$$\frac{10 \text{ mg}}{} \left| \frac{\text{tablet}}{5 \text{ mg}} \right| \frac{10}{5} = 2 \text{ tablets}$$

10. Sequential method:

$$\frac{50 \text{ mg}}{} \left| \frac{\text{mL}}{100 \text{ mg}} \right| \frac{5}{10} = 0.5 \text{ mL}$$

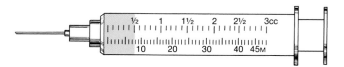

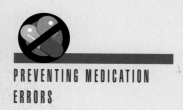

Although medications are ordered by physicians or nurse practitioners and administered by nurses using the "five rights of medication administration," other factors must be considered when administering certain medications or intravenous (IV) fluids.

The **weight** of the patient often must be factored into a medication problem when determining how much medication can safely be given to an infant or a child or an elderly patient.

The dosage of medication available may be in a powdered form that needs **reconstitution** to a liquid form before parenteral or IV administration.

Also, the length of **time** over which medication or IV fluids can be given plays an important role in the safe administration of IV therapy.

To be able to calculate a two-factor–given quantity to one-factor– or two-factor–wanted quantity medication problem, it is important to understand all factors that may need to be considered in some medication problems. With use of dimensional analysis, this chapter will teach you to calculate medication problems involving the weight of the patient, the reconstitution of medications from powder to liquid form, and the amount of time over which medications or IV fluids can be safely administered.

Two-Factor Medication Problems

Outline

MEDICATION PROBLEMS INVOLVING WEIGHT 104

Exercise 5.1: Pediatric Medication Problems Involving Weight 106

MEDICATION PROBLEMS INVOLVING RECONSTITUTION 108

Exercise 5.2: Medication Problems Involving Reconstitution 111

MEDICATION PROBLEMS INVOLVING INTRAVENOUS PUMPS 112

Exercise 5.3: Medication Problems Involving Intravenous Pumps 115

MEDICATION PROBLEMS INVOLVING DROP FACTORS 116

Exercise 5.4: Medication Problems Involving Drop Factors 120

MEDICATION PROBLEMS INVOLVING INTERMITTENT INFUSION 120

Exercise 5.5: Medication Problems Involving Intermittent Infusion 122

Practice Problems for Chapter 5: Two-Factor Medication Problems 124

Post-Test for Chapter 5: Two-Factor Medication Problems 127

Answer Key for Chapter 5: Two-Factor Medication Problems 131

Objectives

After completing this chapter, you will be able to:

1. Solve two-factor–given quantity to one-factor–wanted quantity medication problems involving a specific amount of medication ordered based on the weight of the patient.

2. Calculate medication problems requiring reconstitution of medications by using information from a nursing drug reference, label, or package insert.

3. Solve two-factor–given quantity to two-factor–wanted quantity medication problems involving a specific amount of fluid to be delivered over limited time using an intravenous pump delivering milliliters per hour (mL/hr).

4. Solve two-factor–given quantity to two-factor–wanted quantity medication problems involving a specific amount of fluid to be delivered over a limited time using different types of intravenous tubing that deliver drops per minute (gtt/min) based on a specific *drop factor*.

■ MEDICATION PROBLEMS INVOLVING WEIGHT

When solving problems with dimensional analysis, you can use either the *sequential method* or the *random method* to calculate two-factor–given quantity medication problems. The **given quantity** (the physician's order) contains two parts including a **numerator** (dosage of medication) and a **denominator** (the weight of the patient). This type of medication problem is called a *two-factor* medication problem because the *given quantity* now contains two parts (a numerator and a denominator) instead of just one part (a numerator).

Below is an example of the problem-solving method showing placement of basic terms used in dimensional analysis, applied to a two-factor medication problem involving weight.

Unit Path

Given Quantity	Conversion Factor for Given Quantity (Numerator)	Conversion Factor for Given Quantity (Denominator)		Conversion Computation	Wanted Quantity
2.5 mg	mL	1 kg	60 lb	$2.5 \times 1 \times 6$	15
kg	40 mg	2.2 lb		4.22	8.8

$$= 1.7 \text{ mL}$$

EXAMPLE 5.1

The physician orders gentamicin 2.5 mg/kg IV (intravenous) every 8 hours for infection. The vial of medication is labeled 40 mg/mL. The child weighs 60 lb.

▶ **How many milliliters will you give?**

Given quantity   = 2.5 mg/kg
Wanted quantity = mL
Dose on hand   = 40 mg/mL
Weight   = 60 lb

Sequential method:

STEP 1 Identify the two-factor–given quantity (the physician's order).

Unit Path

Given Quantity	Conversion Factor for Given Quantity (Numerator)	Conversion Factor for Given Quantity (Denominator)	Conversion Computation	Wanted Quantity
2.5 mg				
kg				= mL

STEP 2

Unit Path

Given Quantity	Conversion Factor for Given Quantity (Numerator)	Conversion Factor for Given Quantity (Denominator)	Conversion Computation	Wanted Quantity
2.5 mg	mL			
kg	40 mg			= mL

STEP 3

Unit Path

Given Quantity	Conversion Factor for Given Quantity (Numerator)	Conversion Factor for Given Quantity (Denominator)	Conversion Computation	Wanted Quantity
2.5 ~~mg~~	(mL)	1 ~~kg~~		= mL
~~kg~~	40 ~~mg~~	2.2 lb		

STEP 4

Unit Path

Given Quantity	Conversion Factor for Given Quantity (Numerator)	Conversion Factor for Given Quantity (Denominator)	Conversion Computation	Wanted Quantity
2.5 ~~mg~~	(mL)	1 ~~kg~~ 60 ~~lb~~		= mL
~~kg~~	40 ~~mg~~	2.2 ~~lb~~		

STEP 5

Unit Path

Given Quantity	Conversion Factor for Given Quantity (Numerator)	Conversion Factor for Given Quantity (Denominator)	Conversion Computation	Wanted Quantity
2.5 ~~mg~~	(mL)	1 ~~kg~~ 60 ~~lb~~	$2.5 \times 1 \times 6$ 15	= 1.7 mL
~~kg~~	40 ~~mg~~	2.2 ~~lb~~	4×2.2 8.8	

▶ ▶ ▶ *1.7 mL is the wanted quantity and the answer to the problem.*

Dimensional analysis is a problem-solving method that uses critical thinking. When implementing the *random method* of dimensional analysis, the medication problem can be set up in a number of different ways. The focus is on the correct placement of conversion factors to cancel out all unwanted units. The wanted unit is placed in the numerator to correctly correspond with the wanted quantity.

$$\frac{2.5 \text{ ~~mg~~}}{\text{~~kg~~}} \quad \frac{1 \text{ kg}}{2.2 \text{ ~~lb~~}} \quad \frac{60 \text{ ~~lb~~}}{} \quad \frac{\text{(mL)}}{40 \text{ ~~mg~~}} \quad \frac{2.5 \times 1 \times 6}{2.2 \times 4} \quad \frac{15}{8.8} = 1.7 \text{ mL}$$

PREVENTING MEDICATION ERRORS

One of the most frequent **medication errors** is the error made with the conversion of weight.

The weight conversion [1 kg = 2.2 lb] is often incorrectly written [1 lb = 2.2 kg].

Remember that you would rather tell someone your weight in kilograms as it is a much smaller number [1 kg = 2.2 lb or, put in more realistic terms, 90.9 kg = 200 lb].

Exercise 5.1   **Pediatric Medication Problems Involving Weight**
(See page 131 for answers)

1. Order: furosemide 1 mg/kg IV bid for hypercalcemia. The child weighs 45 lb.

   ▶ **How many milliliters will you give?** _____

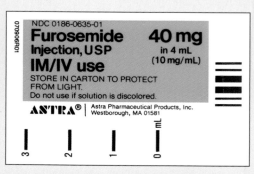

NDC 0186-0635-01

Furosemide
Injection, USP
IM/IV use

40 mg
in 4 mL
(10 mg/mL)

STORE IN CARTON TO PROTECT FROM LIGHT.
Do not use if solution is discolored.

ASTRA® | Astra Pharmaceutical Products, Inc.
Westborough, MA 01581

3   2   1   0 mL

Courtesy of Astra Pharmaceutical Products.

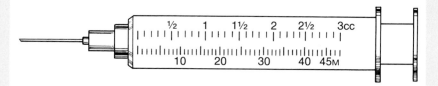

2. Order: atropine sulfate 0.01 mg/kg IV stat for bradycardia. The child weighs 20 lb.

   ▶ **How many milliliters will you give?** _____

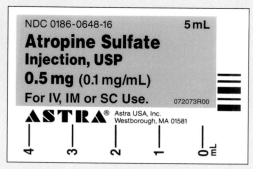

NDC 0186-0648-16   5 mL

Atropine Sulfate
Injection, USP

0.5 mg (0.1 mg/mL)

For IV, IM or SC Use.   072073R00

ASTRA® Astra USA, Inc.
Westborough, MA 01581

4   3   2   1   0 mL

Courtesy of Astra Pharmaceutical Products.

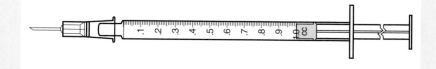

3. Order: phenergan 0.5 mg/kg IV every 4 hours prn for nausea. The
   dose on hand is 25 mg/mL. The child weighs 45 lb.

   ▶ **How many milliliters will you give?** _____

4. Order: morphine 50 mcg/kg IV every 4 hours prn for pain. The child
   weighs 75 lb.

   ▶ **How many milliliters will you give?** _____

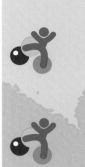

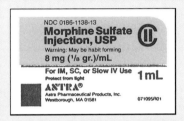

NDC 0186-1138-13
**Morphine Sulfate
Injection, USP**
Warning: May be habit forming
8 mg (¹/₈ gr.)/mL
For IM, SC, or Slow IV Use
Protect from light   **1 mL**
ANTRA®
Astra Pharmaceutical Products, Inc.
Westborough, MA 01581   071095R01

Courtesy of Astra Pharmaceutical Products.

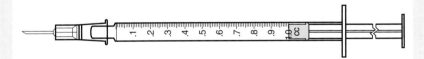

5. Order: Tagamet 10 mg/kg PO qid for prophylaxis of duodenal ulcer.
   The dose on hand is 300 mg/5 mL. The child weighs 70 lb.

   ▶ **How many milliliters will you give?** _____

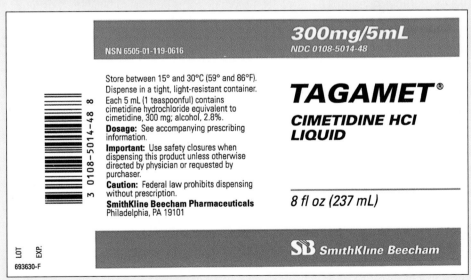

NSN 6505-01-119-0616

300mg/5mL
NDC 0108-5014-48

Store between 15° and 30°C (59° and 86°F).
Dispense in a tight, light-resistant container.
Each 5 mL (1 teaspoonful) contains
cimetidine hydrochloride equivalent to
cimetidine, 300 mg; alcohol, 2.8%.
Dosage: See accompanying prescribing
information.
Important: Use safety closures when
dispensing this product unless otherwise
directed by physician or requested by
purchaser.
Caution: Federal law prohibits dispensing
without prescription.
SmithKline Beecham Pharmaceuticals
Philadelphia, PA 19101

TAGAMET®

**CIMETIDINE HCl
LIQUID**

8 fl oz (237 mL)

SB SmithKline Beecham

LOT   EXP.
693630-F

Courtesy of SmithKline Beecham Pharmaceuticals.

(Exercise continues on page 108)

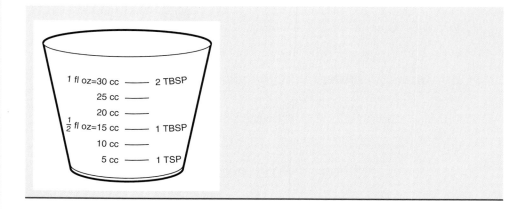

■ MEDICATION PROBLEMS INVOLVING RECONSTITUTION

Some medications in vials are in a powder form and need reconstitution before administration. **Reconstitution** involves adding a specific amount of sterile solution (also called **diluent**) to the vial to change the powder to a liquid form. Information on how much diluent to add to the vial and what dosage of medication per milliliter will result after reconstitution (also called **yield**) can be obtained from a nursing drug reference, label, or package insert.

EXAMPLE 5.2

The physician orders Mezlin (mezlocillin) 50 mg/kg every 4 hours IV for infection. The child weighs 60 lb. The pharmacy sends a vial of medication labeled Mezlin 1 g. The nursing drug reference provides information to reconstitute 1 g of medication with 10 mL of sterile water for injection, 0.9% NaCl, or D5W.

▶ **How many milliliters will you draw from the vial?**

Given quantity   = 50 mg/kg
Wanted quantity = mL
Dose on hand   = 1 g/10 mL (yields 1 g/10 mL)
Weight   = 60 lb

Random method:

Unit Path

Given Quantity	Conversion Factor for Given Quantity (Numerator)		Conversion Factor for Given Quantity (Denominator)		Conversion Computation		Wanted Quantity
50 mg	1 kg	60 lb	10 (mL)	1 g	5 × 1 × 6 × 1	30	13.63 mL
kg	2.2 lb		1 g	1000 mg	2.2	2.2	or 13.6 mL

$= $ 13.63 mL or 13.6 mL

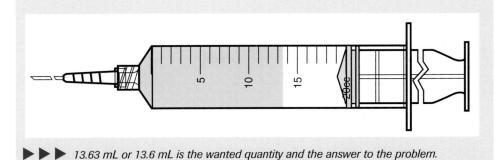

▶ ▶ ▶ *13.63 mL or 13.6 mL is the wanted quantity and the answer to the problem.*

EXAMPLE 5.3

Order: Solu-Medrol 40 mg IV every 4 hours for inflammation.

▶ How many milliliters will you draw from the vial?

Solu-Medrol®   **Upjohn**

brand of methylprednisolone sodium succinate sterile powder
(methylprednisolone sodium succinate for injection, USP)

For Intravenous or Intramuscular Administration

125 mg Act-O-Vial System (Single-Dose Vial)—Each 2 mL (when mixed) contains methylprednisolone sodium succinate equivalent to 125 mg methylprednisolone; also 1.6 mg
monobasic sodium phosphate anhydrous; 17.4 mg dibasic sodium phosphate dried; 17.6 mg
benzyl alcohol added as preservative

DOSAGE AND ADMINISTRATION
   When high dose therapy is desired, the recommended dose of SOLU-MEDROL Sterile
Powder is 30 mg/kg administered intravenously over at least 30 minutes. This dose may be
repeated every 4 to 6 hours for 48 hours.
   In general, high dose corticosteroid therapy should be continued only until the patient's
condition has stabilized; usually not beyond 48 to 72 hours.
   Although adverse effects associated with high dose short-term corticoid therapy are
uncommon, peptic ulceration may occur. Prophylactic antacid therapy may be indicated.
   In other indications initial dosage will vary from 10 to 40 mg of methylprednisolone depend-
ing on the clinical problem being treated. The larger doses may be required for short-term
management of severe, acute conditions. The initial dose usually should be given intravenously over a period of several minutes. Subsequent doses may be given intravenously or
intramuscularly at intervals dictated by the patient's response and clinical condition. Corticoid
therapy is an adjunct to, and not replacement for conventional therapy.
   Dosage may be reduced for infants and children but should be governed more by the
severity of the condition and response of the patient than by age or size. It should not be less
than 0.5 mg per kg every 24 hours.
   Dosage must be decreased or discontinued gradually when the drug has been administered for more than a few days. If a period of spontaneous remission occurs in a chronic condition, treatment should be discontinued. Routine laboratory studies, such as urinalysis, two-
hour postprandial blood sugar, determination of blood pressure and body weight, and a chest
X-ray should be made at regular intervals during prolonged therapy. Upper GI X-rays are
desirable in patients with an ulcer history or significant dyspepsia.
   SOLU-MEDROL may be administered by intravenous or intramuscular injection or by intravenous infusion, the preferred method for initial emergency use being intravenous injection.
To administer by intravenous (or intramuscular) injection, prepare solution as directed. The
desired dose may be administered intravenously over a period of several minutes. If desired,
the medication may be administered in diluted solutions by adding Water for Injection or
other suitable diluent (see below) to the **Act-O-Vial** and withdrawing the indicated dose.
   To prepare solutions for intravenous infusion, first prepare the solution for injection as
directed. This solution may then be added to indicated amounts of 5% dextrose in water, isotonic saline solution or 5% dextrose in isotonic saline solution.

Multiple Sclerosis
In treatment of acute exacerbations of multiple sclerosis, daily doses of 200 mg of prednisolone for a week followed by 80 mg every other day for 1 month have been shown to be
effective (4 mg of methylprednisolone is equivalent to 5 mg of prednisolone).

DIRECTIONS FOR USING THE ACT-O-VIAL SYSTEM
1. Press down on plastic activator to force diluent into the
   lower compartment.
2. Gently agitate to effect solution.
3. Remove plastic tab covering center of stopper.
4. Sterilize top of stopper with a suitable germicide.
5. Insert needle **squarely through center** of stopper
   until tip is just visible. Invert vial and withdraw dose.

STORAGE CONDITIONS
   Store unreconstituted product at controlled room temperature 15° to 30° C (59° to 86° F).
   Store solution at controlled room temperature 15° to 30° C (59° to 86° F).
   Use solution within 48 hours after mixing.

HOW SUPPLIED
   SOLU-MEDROL Sterile Powder is available in the following packages:
40 mg Act-O-Vial System (Single-Dose Vial)   **500 mg** Vial NDC 0009-0758-01
   1 mL NDC 0009-0113-12   **500 mg** Vial with Diluent NDC 0009-0887-01
   25—1 mL NDC 0009-0113-13   **500 mg Act-O-Vial System (Single-Dose Vial)**
   25—1 mL NDC 0009-0113-19   4 mL NDC 0009-0765-02
125 mg Act-O-Vial System (Single-Dose Vial)   **1 gram** Vial NDC 0009-0698-01
   2 mL NDC 0009-0190-09   **1 gram Act-O-Vial System (Single-Dose Vial)**
   25—2 mL NDC 0009-0190-10   8 mL NDC 0009-3389-01
   25—2 mL NDC 0009-0190-16   **2 gram** Vial NDC 0009-0988-01
                                                    2 gram Vial with Diluent NDC 0009-0796-01

Courtesy of the Upjohn Company.

(Example continues on page 110)

Given quantity   = 40 mg
Wanted quantity = mL
Dose on hand   = 125 mg/2 mL (yield from 2 mL Act-O-Vial)

Sequential method:

$$\frac{40 \text{ mg}}{} \quad \frac{2 \text{ mL}}{125 \text{ mg}} \quad \frac{40 \times 2}{125} \quad \frac{80}{125} = 0.64 \text{ mL or } 0.6 \text{ mL}$$

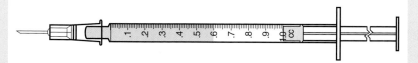

▶▶▶ *0.6 mL is the wanted quantity and the answer to the problem.*

EXAMPLE 5.4

Order: Claforan 50 mg/kg IV every 8 hours for infection. The infant weighs 12 kg.

▶ **How many milliliters will you draw from the vial after reconstitution?**

719000-2/95

Claforan®

Sterile (sterile cefotaxime sodium)
and
Injection (cefotaxime sodium injection)

HOECHST-ROUSSEL
Pharmaceuticals Incorporated
Somerville, NJ 08876-1258
REG TM HOECHST AG

Neonates, Infants, and Children
The following dosage schedule is recommended:

Neonates (birth to 1 month):
    0-1 week of age   50 mg/kg per dose every 12 hours IV
    1-4 weeks of age   50 mg/kg per dose every 8 hours IV
It is not necessary to differentiate between premature and normal-gestational age infants.
Infants and Children (1 month to 12 years): For body weights less than 50 kg, the recommended daily dose is 50 to 180 mg/kg IM or IV body weight divided into four to six equal doses. The higher dosages should be used for more severe or serious infections, including meningitis. For body weights 50 kg or more, the usual adult dosage should be used; the maximum daily dosage should not exceed 12 grams.

Courtesy of Hoechst-Roussel Pharmaceuticals.

Supply: Claforan 1 g/10 mL
The package insert states: Reconstitute vials with at least 10 mL of sterile water for injection.

Given quantity   = 50 mg/kg
Wanted quantity = mL
Dose on hand   = 1 g/10 mL
Weight   = 12 kg

Random method:

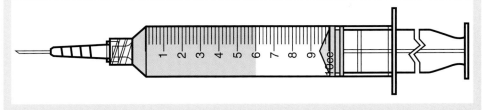

$$\frac{50 \text{ mg}}{\text{kg}} \mid \frac{10 \text{ mL}}{1 \text{ g}} \mid \frac{1 \text{ g}}{1000 \text{ mg}} \mid 12 \text{ kg} \mid \frac{5 \times 1 \times 1 \times 12}{1 \times 10} \mid \frac{60}{10} = 6 \text{ mL}$$

▶▶▶ *6 mL is the wanted quantity and the answer to the problem.*

Exercise 5.2	**Medication Problems Involving Reconstitution**
	(See pages 131–132 for answers)

1. Order: Ancef 500 mg IV every 8 hours for infection.

   ▶ **How many milliliters will you draw out of the vial after reconstitution?** _____

   (Ancef is reconstituted using 50 mL sodium chloride.)

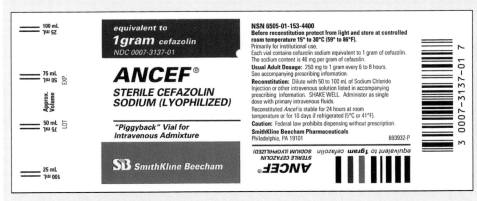

Courtesy of SmithKline Beecham Pharmaceuticals.

2. Order: Primaxin 250 mg IV every 6 hours for infection

   Supply: Primaxin vial labeled 500 mg. Reconstitute with 10 mL of compatible diluent and shake well.

   ▶ **How many milliliters will you draw from the vial after reconstitution?** _____

(Exercise continues on page 112)

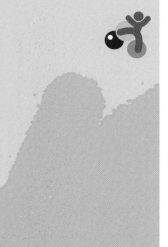

3. Order: Unasyn (ampicillin) 50 mg/kg IV every 4 hours for infection

   Supply: Unasyn 1.5-g vial

   Nursing drug reference: Reconstitute each Unasyn 1.5-g vial with 4 mL of sterile water to yield 375 mg/mL.

   The child weighs 40 kg.

   ▶ **How many milliliters will you draw from the vial after reconstitution?** _____

4. Order: erythromycin 750 mg IV every 6 hours for infection

   Supply: erythromycin 1-g vial labeled: Reconstitute with 20 mL of sterile water for injection.

   ▶ **How many milliliters will you draw from the vial after reconstitution?** _____

5. Order: Fortaz 30 mg/kg IV every 8 hours for infection

   Supply: Fortaz 500-mg vial labeled: Reconstitute with 5 mL of sterile water for injection

   The child weighs 65 lb.

   ▶ **How many milliliters will you draw from the vial after reconstitution?** _____

PREVENTING MEDICATION ERRORS

When administering IV medications and fluids, always check a nursing drug reference to obtain the correct information regarding how much medication or fluid can safely be administered to prevent **medication errors.**

It is the responsibility of the nurse to be familiar with the different types of IV pumps that are used to deliver IV medications or fluids. All medications delivered by the IV route should be delivered using an IV pump to ensure accuracy and safety of delivery.

■ MEDICATION PROBLEMS INVOLVING INTRAVENOUS PUMPS

IV medications are administered by drawing a specific amount of medication from a vial or ampule and inserting that medication into an existing IV line. All IV medications must be given with specific thought to exactly how much *time* it should take to administer the medication. Information regarding time may be obtained from a nursing drug reference, label, or package insert, or may be specifically ordered by the physician.

Although IV medications can be administered IV push, the time involved often requires the use of an IV pump. All IV pumps deliver milliliters per hour (mL/hr or cc/hr) but may vary in operational capacity or size.

Below is an example of the dimensional analysis problem-solving method with basic terms applied to a medication problem involving an IV pump.

Unit Path

Given Quantity	Conversion Factor for Given Quantity (Numerator)	Conversion Computation	Wanted Quantity
$\dfrac{1500 \text{ Units}}{\text{hr}}$	$\dfrac{250 \text{ mL}}{25{,}000 \text{ Units}}$	$\dfrac{15}{\text{hr}}$	$= 15 \text{ mL}$

EXAMPLE 5.5

The physician orders heparin 1500 units/hr IV. The pharmacy sends an IV bag labeled: Heparin 25,000 units in 250 mL of D5W.

▶ **Calculate the IV pump setting for milliliters per hour.**

Given quantity   = 1500 units/hr
Wanted quantity = mL/hr
Dose on hand   = 25,000 units/250 mL

Sequential method:

STEP 1 **Begin by identifying the given quantity. Establish the unit path to the wanted quantity.**

Unit Path

Given Quantity	Conversion Factor for Given Quantity (Numerator)	Conversion Computation	Wanted Quantity
$\dfrac{1500 \text{ Units}}{\text{hr}}$			$= \dfrac{\text{mL}}{\text{hr}}$

STEP 2

Unit Path

Given Quantity	Conversion Factor for Given Quantity (Numerator)	Conversion Computation	Wanted Quantity
$\dfrac{1500 \text{ Units}}{\text{hr}}$	$\dfrac{250 \text{ mL}}{25{,}000 \text{ Units}}$		$= \dfrac{\text{mL}}{\text{hr}}$

STEP 3

Unit Path

Given Quantity	Conversion Factor for Given Quantity (Numerator)	Conversion Computation	Wanted Quantity
$\dfrac{1500 \text{ Units}}{\text{hr}}$	$\dfrac{250 \text{ mL}}{25{,}000 \text{ Units}}$	15	$= \dfrac{15 \text{ mL}}{\text{hr}}$

▶▶▶ *15 mL/hr is the wanted quantity and the answer to the problem.*

THINKING IT THROUGH

The two-factor–given quantity (the physician's order) contains a **numerator** (the dosage of medication) and a **denominator** (time). The wanted quantity (the answer to the problem) also contains a numerator (mL) and a denominator (time). This is called a two-factor–given quantity to a two-factor–wanted quantity medication problem. The denominator of the given quantity (hr) corresponds with the denominator of the wanted quantity (hr); therefore, only the numerator of the given quantity (units) needs to be canceled from the problem.

After factoring in the dose on hand, the unwanted unit (units) is canceled from the problem and the wanted unit (mL) remains in the numerator to correspond with the wanted quantity. The same number values are canceled from the numerator and denominator, leaving 15 mL/hr.

THINKING IT THROUGH

In this problem, the needed two factors are already identified in the given quantity and, therefore, require no additional conversions. The 20 mEq of KCl added to the IV bag is included as part of the 500 mL and is additional information for the nurse, but not part of the calculation.

EXAMPLE 5.6

The physician orders 500 mL of 0.45% NS with 20 mEq of KCl to infuse over 8 hours.

▶ **Calculate the number of milliliters per hour to set the IV pump.**

Given quantity   = 500 mL/8 hr
Wanted quantity = mL/hr

Sequential method:

$$\frac{500 \; \cancel{mL}}{8 \; \cancel{hr}} \; \bigg| \; \frac{500}{8} = \frac{62.5 \; mL}{} \; or \; \frac{63 \; mL}{hr}$$

▶▶▶ *63 mL/hr is the wanted quantity and the answer to the problem.*

THINKING IT THROUGH

The given quantity has been identified as what the physician orders, but also can be information that the nurse has obtained. The nurse may know that the IV pump is set to deliver 11 mL/hr, but wants to know if the dosage of medication the patient is receiving is within a safe dosage range.

EXAMPLE 5.7

The physician orders aminophylline 44 mg/hr IV. The pharmacy sends an IV bag labeled: Aminophylline 1 g/250 mL NS.

▶ **Calculate the milliliters per hour to set the IV pump.**

Given quantity   = 44 mg/hr
Wanted quantity = mL/hr
Dose on hand   = 1 g/250 mL

Random method:

$$\frac{44 \; \cancel{mg}}{\cancel{hr}} \; \bigg| \; \frac{250 \; \cancel{mL}}{1 \; \cancel{g}} \; \bigg| \; \frac{1 \; \cancel{g}}{1000 \; \cancel{mg}} \; \bigg| \; \frac{44 \times 25}{100} \; \bigg| \; \frac{1100}{100} = \frac{11 \; mL}{hr}$$

▶▶▶ *11 mL/hr is the wanted quantity and the answer to the problem.*

THINKING IT THROUGH

The dose on hand is factored in and allows the unwanted unit (mL) to be canceled.

EXAMPLE 5.8

The nurse checks the IV pump and documents that the pump is set at and delivering 11 mL/hr and that the IV bag hanging is labeled: Aminophylline 1 g/250 mL.

▶ **How many milligrams per hour is the patient receiving?**

Given quantity   = 11 mL/hr
Wanted quantity = mg/hr
Dose on hand   = 1 g/250 mL

Sequential method:

STEP 1

$$\frac{11 \text{ mL}}{\text{hr}} \bigg| = \frac{\text{mg}}{\text{hr}}$$

STEP 2

$$\frac{11 \text{ mL}}{\text{hr}} \bigg| \frac{1 \text{ g}}{250 \text{ mL}} = \frac{\text{mg}}{\text{hr}}$$

STEP 3

$$\frac{11 \text{ mL}}{\text{hr}} \bigg| \frac{1 \text{ g}}{250 \text{ mL}} \bigg| \frac{1000 \text{ mg}}{1 \text{ g}} \bigg| \frac{11 \times 100}{25} \bigg| \frac{1100}{25} = \frac{44 \text{ mg}}{\text{hr}}$$

▶▶▶ *44 mg/hr is the wanted quantity and the answer to the problem.*

Exercise 5.3	**Medication Problems Involving Intravenous Pumps**

(See page 132 for answers)

1. Order: heparin 1800 units/hr IV

   Supply: heparin 25,000 units/250 mL D5W

   ▶ **Calculate the milliliters per hour to set the IV pump.** _____

2. Order: aminophylline 35 mg/hr IV

   Supply: aminophylline 1 g/250 mL NS

   ▶ **Calculate the milliliters per hour to set the IV pump.** _____

3. Information obtained by the nurse: heparin 25,000 units in 250 mL D5W is infusing at 30 mL/hr.

   ▶ **How many units per hour is the patient receiving?** _____

(Exercise continues on page 116)

4. Information obtained by the nurse: aminophylline 1 g/250 mL NS is infusing at 15 mL/hr.

   ▶ **How many milligrams per hour is the patient receiving?** _____

5. Order: heparin 900 units/hr IV

   Supply: heparin 25,000 units/500 mL D5W

   ▶ **Calculate the milliliters per hour to set the IV pump.** _____

PREVENTING MEDICATION ERRORS

When IV fluids are administered by gravity (without the use of an IV pump), it is the responsibility of the nurse to investigate the history of each patient to ensure safe delivery of IV fluids.

IV fluids that flow by gravity need to be monitored closely because the flow of the fluids can change with the position of the hand or arm. Some patients with a history of congestive heart failure do not tolerate large volumes of IV fluids.

■ MEDICATION PROBLEMS INVOLVING DROP FACTORS

Although IV pumps are used whenever possible, there are situations (no IV pumps available) and circumstances (outpatient or home care) that arise when IV pumps are not available and IV fluids or medications might be administered using gravity flow. **Gravity flow** involves calculating the drops per minute (gtt/min) required to infuse IV fluids or medications. When IV fluids or medications are administered using gravity flow, it is important to know the drop factor for the IV tubing that is being used. **Drop factor** is the drops per milliliter (gtt/mL) that the IV tubing will produce. Two types of IV tubing are available for gravity flow. *Macrotubing* delivers a large drop and is available in 10 gtt/mL, 15 gtt/mL, and 20 gtt/mL (Table 5.1); and *microtubing* delivers a small drop and is available in 60 gtt/mL.

Regardless of the IV tubing used, the problem can be solved by dimensional analysis. Below is an example of a medication problem involving drop factors using the dimensional analysis method.

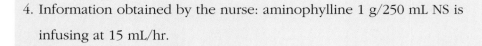

Unit Path

Given Quantity	Conversion Factor for Given Quantity (Numerator)	Conversion Computation	Wanted Quantity		
$\dfrac{250\ \text{mL}}{30\ \text{min}}$	$\dfrac{10\ \text{gtt}}{\text{mL}}$	$\dfrac{250 \times 1}{3}$	$\dfrac{250}{3} =$	$\dfrac{83.3\ \text{gtt}}{\text{min}}$ or	$\dfrac{83\ \text{gtt}}{\text{min}}$

■ TABLE 5.1	Examples of Different Macrodrip Factors
MANUFACTURER	**DROPS PER MILLILITER (GTT/ML)**
Travenol	10
Abbott	15
McGaw	15
Cutter	20

EXAMPLE 5.9

The physician orders 250 mL of normal saline to infuse in 30 minutes. The drop factor listed on the IV tubing box is 10 gtt/mL.

▶ **Calculate the number of drops per minute required to infuse the IV bolus.**

Given quantity   = 250 mL/30 min
Wanted quantity = gtt/min
Drop factor   = 10 gtt/mL

Sequential method:

STEP 1 **Begin by identifying the given quantity and establishing a unit path to the wanted quantity.**

	Unit Path		
Given Quantity	**Conversion Factor for Given Quantity (Numerator)**	**Conversion Computation**	**Wanted Quantity**
$\dfrac{250 \text{ mL}}{30 \text{ min}}$			$= \dfrac{\text{gtt}}{\text{min}}$

STEP 2

	Unit Path		
Given Quantity	**Conversion Factor for Given Quantity (Numerator)**	**Conversion Computation**	**Wanted Quantity**
$\dfrac{250 \text{ mL}}{30 \text{ min}}$	$\dfrac{10 \text{ gtt}}{\text{mL}}$		$= \dfrac{\text{gtt}}{\text{min}}$

STEP 3

	Unit Path				
Given Quantity	**Conversion Factor for Given Quantity (Numerator)**	**Conversion Computation**	**Wanted Quantity**		
$\dfrac{250 \text{ mL}}{30 \text{ min}}$	$\dfrac{10 \text{ gtt}}{\text{mL}}$	$\dfrac{250 \times 1}{3}$	$\dfrac{250}{3} =$	$\dfrac{83.3 \text{ gtt}}{\text{min}}$ or	$\dfrac{83 \text{ gtt}}{\text{min}}$

▶▶▶ *83 gtt is the wanted quantity and the answer to the problem.*

THINKING IT THROUGH

The unwanted unit (mL) is canceled, and the wanted unit (gtt) is placed in the numerator. Another unwanted unit (hr) needs to be canceled from the unit path.

The conversion factor (1 hr = 60 min) has been factored in to allow the unwanted unit (hr) to be canceled and the wanted unit (min) is placed in the denominator.

EXAMPLE 5.10

In some situations (home care), it may be important for the nurse to know exactly how long a specific amount of IV fluid will take to infuse. The physician may order a limited amount of IV fluid to infuse at a specific number of drops per minute (gtt/min).

The physician orders 1000 mL of D5W and 0.45% NS to infuse over 8 hours. The drop factor is 20 gtt/mL.

▶ **Calculate the number of drops per minute required to infuse the IV volume.**

Given quantity   = 1000 mL/8 hr
Wanted quantity = gtt/min
Drop factor   = 20 gtt/mL

Sequential method:

STEP 1

$$\frac{1000 \text{ mL}}{8 \text{ hr}} \left| \frac{20 \text{ gtt}}{\text{mL}} \right. = \frac{\text{gtt}}{\text{min}}$$

STEP 2

$$\frac{1000 \text{ mL}}{8 \text{ hr}} \left| \frac{20 \text{ gtt}}{\text{mL}} \right| \frac{1 \text{ hr}}{60 \text{ min}} = \frac{\text{gtt}}{\text{min}}$$

STEP 3

$$\frac{1000 \text{ mL}}{8 \text{ hr}} \left| \frac{20 \text{ gtt}}{\text{mL}} \right| \frac{1 \text{ hr}}{60 \text{ min}} \left| \frac{1000 \times 2 \times 1}{8 \times 6} \right| \frac{2000}{48} = \frac{41.66 \text{ gtt}}{\text{min}}$$

$$\frac{41.66 \text{ gtt}}{\text{min}} \text{ or } \frac{42 \text{ gtt}}{\text{min}}$$

▶▶▶ *42 gtt/min is the wanted quantity and the answer to the problem.*

EXAMPLE 5.11

It is safe nursing practice to monitor an infusing IV every 2 hours to make sure it is infusing without difficulty and on time. It may be necessary to hang the next IV after $7\frac{1}{2}$ hours (before the estimated completion time) to keep the IV from running dry.

The physician orders 1000 mL of D5W. The drop factor is 10 gtt/mL. The infusion is dripping at 21 gtt/min.

▶ **How many hours will it take for the IV to infuse?**

Given quantity = 1000 mL
Wanted quantity = hr
Drop factor = 10 gtt/mL

STEP 1

$$\frac{1000 \text{ mL}}{\quad} = \text{hr}$$

STEP 2

$$\frac{1000 \text{ mL}}{} \left| \frac{10 \text{ gtt}}{\text{mL}} \right. = \text{hr}$$

STEP 3

$$\frac{1000 \text{ mL}}{} \left| \frac{10 \text{ gtt}}{\text{mL}} \right| \frac{\text{min}}{21 \text{ gtt}} = \text{hr}$$

STEP 4

$$\frac{1000 \text{ mL}}{} \left| \frac{10 \text{ gtt}}{\text{mL}} \right| \frac{\text{min}}{21 \text{ gtt}} \left| \frac{1 \text{ hr}}{60 \text{ min}} \right. = \text{hr}$$

STEP 5

$$\frac{1000 \text{ mL}}{} \left| \frac{10 \text{ gtt}}{\text{mL}} \right| \frac{\text{min}}{21 \text{ gtt}} \left| \frac{1 \text{ hr}}{60 \text{ min}} \right| \frac{1000 \times 1 \times 1}{21 \times 6} = \frac{1000}{126} = 7.93 \text{ hr or } 7.9 \text{ hr}$$

▶ ▶ ▶ *8 hours is the wanted quantity and the answer to the problem.*

| **Exercise 5.4** | **Medication Problems Involving Drop Factors** |

(See page 132 for answers)

1. Order: 800 mL D5W to infuse in 8 hours

   Drop factor: 15 gtt/mL

   ▶ **Calculate the number of drops per minute.** _____

2. Order: Infuse 250 mL NS

   Drop factor: 15 gtt/mL

   Infusion rate: 60 gtt/min

   ▶ **Calculate the hours to infuse.** _____

3. Order: 150 mL over 60 minutes

   Drop factor: 10 gtt/mL

   ▶ **Calculate the number of drops per minute.** _____

4. Order: 1000 mL D5W/0.9% NS

   Drop factor: 15 gtt/mL

   Infusion rate: 50 gtt/min

   ▶ **Calculate the number of hours to infuse.** _____

5. Order: 500 mL over 4 hours

   Drop factor: 15 gtt/mL

   ▶ **Calculate the number of drops per minute.** _____

PREVENTING MEDICATION ERRORS

When adding reconstituted medications to an IV solution, always check a nursing drug reference for compatibility of the solutions. To prevent precipitation and/or avoid extravasations, certain medications must be mixed in certain fluids and then further diluted.

Example: **Dilantin**® (phenytoin) must be reconstituted with normal saline (0.9% NaCl) and **never** administered into an IV line of dextrose in water (D_5W). Dilantin may only be further diluted with normal saline (0.9% NaCl).

Example: **Erythromycin** must be reconstituted with sterile water and may be further diluted in normal saline (0.9% NaCl) or dextrose in water (D_5W).

Example: **Acyclovir** must be reconstituted with sterile water and further diluted in varying strengths and combinations of normal saline (0.9% NaCl) and dextrose in water (D_5W).

■ MEDICATION PROBLEMS INVOLVING INTERMITTENT INFUSION

IV medications can be delivered over a specific amount of time by *intermittent infusion*. These medications require the use of an infusion pump. Some must be reconstituted and further diluted in a specific type and amount of IV fluid and delivered over a limited time. Others do not need to be reconstituted, but must be further diluted in a specific type and amount of IV fluid and delivered over a limited time.

EXAMPLE 5.12

The physician ordered erythromycin 500 mg IV every 6 hours for infection. The pharmacy sends a vial labeled: Erythromycin 1 g. The nursing drug reference provides information to reconstitute 1 g of erythromycin with 20 mL of sterile water and further dilute in 250 mL of 0.9% NS and to infuse over 1 hour.

▶ **How many milliliters will you draw from the vial after reconstitution?**

▶ **Calculate the milliliters per hour to set the IV pump.**

This order contains two problems. The first involves how many milliliters to draw from the vial after reconstitution, and the second involves how many milliliters per hour to set the IV pump.

STEP 1

▶ **How many milliliters will you draw from the vial after reconstitution?**

Given quantity = 500 mg
Wanted quantity = mL
Dose on hand = 1 g/20 mL

Random method:

$$\frac{500\ \text{mg}}{} \left| \frac{20\ \text{mL}}{1\ \text{g}} \right| \frac{1\ \text{g}}{1000\ \text{mg}} \left| \frac{5 \times 2}{1} \right| \frac{10}{1} = 10\ \text{mL}$$

▶▶▶ *The wanted quantity is 10 mL, and is the amount that will need to be drawn from the vial and added to the 250 mL of 0.9% NS. After adding the 10 mL to the IV bag, the IV bag will now contain 260 mL.*

STEP 2

▶ **Calculate the milliliters per hour to set the IV pump.**

Given quantity = 260 mL/1 hr
Wanted quantity = mL/hr

Sequential method:

$$\frac{260\ \text{mL}}{1\ \text{hr}} \left| \frac{260}{1} \right| = \frac{260\ \text{mL}}{\text{hr}}$$

▶▶▶ *The IV pump is set at 260 mL/hr to infuse the 500 mg of erythromycin ordered by the physician.*

(Example continues on page 122)

STEP 2 (alternative): If an IV pump was unavailable, the infusion could be delivered by gravity using IV tubing with a drop factor of 10 gtt/mL.

▶ **Calculate the drops per minute required to infuse the IV volume.**

Given quantity   = 260 mL/1 hr
Wanted quantity = gtt/min
Drop factor   = 10 gtt/mL

Sequential method:

$$\frac{260 \ \text{mL}}{1 \ \text{hr}} \ \Bigg| \ \frac{10 \ \text{gtt}}{\text{mL}} \ \Bigg| \ \frac{1 \ \text{hr}}{60 \ \text{min}} \ \Bigg| \ \frac{260 \times 1 \times 1}{1 \times 6} \ \Bigg| \ \frac{260}{6} = \frac{43.3 \ \text{or} \ 43 \ \text{gtt}}{\text{min}}$$

Exercise 5.5   **Medication Problems Involving Intermittent Infusion**
(See pages 132–133 for answers)

1. Order: ampicillin 250 mg IV every 4 hours for infection

   Supply: ampicillin 1-g vial

   Nursing drug reference: Reconstitute with 10 mL of 0.9% NS and further dilute in 50 mL NS. Infuse over 15 min.

   ▶ **How many milliliters will you draw from the vial after reconstitution?** _____

   ▶ **Calculate the milliliters per hour to set the IV pump.** _____

   ▶ **Calculate the drops per minute with a drop factor of 10 gtt/mL.** _____

2. Order: clindamycin 0.3 g IV every 6 hours for infection

   Supply: clindamycin 600 mg/4-mL vial

   Nursing drug reference: Dilute with 50 mL 0.9% NS and infuse over 15 min.

   ▶ **How many milliliters will you draw from the vial?** _____

   ▶ **Calculate the milliliters per hour to set the IV pump.** _____

   ▶ **Calculate the drops per minute with a drop factor of 15 gtt/mL.** _____

3. Order: Mezlin 3 g IV every 4 hours for infection

   Supply: Mezlin 4-g vial

   Nursing drug reference: Reconstitute each 1-g vial with 10 mL of 0.9%

   NS and further dilute in 100 mL 0.9% NS to infuse over 1 hr.

   ▶ **How many milliliters will you draw from the vial after reconstitution?** _____

   ▶ **Calculate the milliliters per hour to set the IV pump.** _____

   ▶ **Calculate the drops per minute with a drop factor of 20 gtt/mL.** _____

4. Order: Unasyn 1000 mg IV every 6 hours for infection

   Supply: Unasyn 1.5-g vial

   Nursing drug reference: Reconstitute with 4 mL of 0.9% NS and further

   dilute with 100 mL NS to infuse over 1 hr.

   ▶ **How many milliliters will you draw from the vial after reconstitution?** _____

   ▶ **Calculate the milliliters per hour to set the IV pump.** _____

   ▶ **Calculate the drops per minute with a drop factor of 20 gtt/mL.** _____

5. Order: Zantac 50 mg IV every 6 hours for ulcers

   Supply: Zantac 25-mg/mL vial

   Nursing drug reference: Dilute with 50 mL 0.9% NS to infuse over 30 min.

   ▶ **How many milliliters will you draw from the vial?** _____

   ▶ **Calculate the milliliters per hour to set the IV pump.** _____

   ▶ **Calculate the drops per minute with a drop factor of 10 gtt/mL.** _____

S U M M A R Y

This chapter has taught you to calculate two-factor medication problems involving the weight of the patient, reconstitution of medications, and the amount of time over which medications and intravenous fluids can be safely administered. To demonstrate your ability to calculate medication problems accurately, complete the following practice problems.

Practice Problems for Chapter 5	**Two-Factor Medication Problems**

(See pages 133–134 for answers)

1. Order: verapamil 0.2 mg/kg IV for arrhythmia

   Supply: verapamil (Isoptin) 5 mg/2 mL

   Child's weight: 10 lb

   ▶ **How many milliliters will you give?** _____

2. Order: Tylenol Elixir 10 mg/kg every 4 hours prn for fever

   Supply: Tylenol Elixir 160 mg/5 mL

   Child's weight: 8 kg

   ▶ **How many milliliters will you give?** _____

3. Order: Fortaz 1.25 g IV every 8 hours for infection

   Supply: Fortaz 2-g vial

   Nursing drug reference: Dilute each 2 g with 10 mL sterile water for injection.

   ▶ **How many milliliters will you draw from the vial after reconstitution?** _____

4. Order: Unasyn 750 mg IV every 8 hours for infection

   Supply: Unasyn 1.5-g vial

   Nursing drug reference: Reconstitute with 4 mL of sterile water for injection.

   ▶ **How many milliliters will you draw from the vial after reconstitution?** _____

5. Order: heparin 700 units/hr for anticoagulation

   Supply: heparin 25,000 units/250 mL NS

   ▶ **At how many milliliters per hour will you set the IV pump?** _____

6. Information obtained by the nurse: Zantac 150 mg in 250 mL NS is infusing at 11 mL/hr.

   ▶ **How many milligrams per hour is the patient receiving?** _____

7. Order: 1000 mL D5W/0.9% NS to infuse over 8 hours

   Drop factor: 20 gtt/mL

   ▶ **Calculate the number of drops per minute.** _____

8. Order: Infuse 750 mL NS

   Drop factor: 15 gtt/mL

   Infusion rate: 18 gtt/min

   ▶ **Calculate the number of hours to infuse.** _____

9. Order: vancomycin 10 mg/kg IV every 8 hours for infection

   Supply: vancomycin 500-mg vial

   Infant's weight: 20 lb

   Nursing drug reference: Dilute each 500-mg vial with 10 mL of sterile

   water for injection and further dilute in 100 mL of 0.9% NS to infuse

   over 1 hr.

   ▶ **How many milliliters will you draw from the vial after**
      reconstitution? _____

   ▶ **Calculate the milliliters per hour to set the**
      IV pump. _____

   ▶ **Calculate the drops per minute with a drop factor of**
      10 gtt/mL. _____

10. Order: acyclovir 355 mg IV every 8 hours for herpes

    Supply: acyclovir 500-mg vial

    Nursing drug reference: Reconstitute each 500 mg with 10 mL of sterile

    water for injection and further dilute in 100 mL NS to infuse over 1 hr.

    ▶ **How many milliliters will you draw from the vial after**
       reconstitution? _____

    ▶ **Calculate the milliliters per hour to set the**
       IV pump. _____

    ▶ **Calculate the drops per minute with a drop factor of**
       20 gtt/mL. _____

Chapter 5 Post-Test: Two-Factor Medication Problems

Name _____   **Date** _____

1. Order: Furosemide 2 mg/kg PO every 8 hours for congestive heart failure

   The child weighs 10 kg.

   ▶ **How many milliliters will you give?** _____

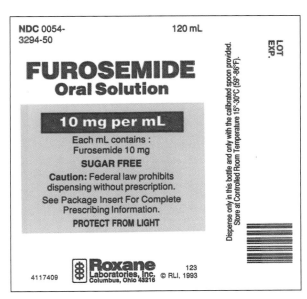

Courtesy of Roxane Laboratories.

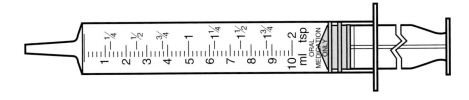

2. Order: meperidine 1.5 mg/kg PO every 4 hours for pain

   The child weighs 22 lb.

   ▶ **How many milliliters will you give?** _____

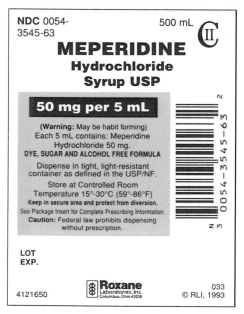

Courtesy of Roxane Laboratories.

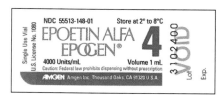

3. Order: Epogen 100 units/kg IV tid for anemia secondary to chronic renal failure

   The patient weighs 160 lb.

   ▶ **How many milliliters will you give?** _____

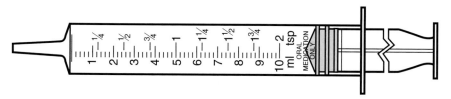

Courtesy of Amgen, Inc.

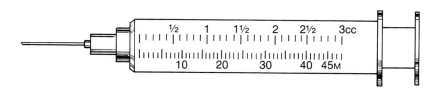

4. Order: Augmentin 10 mg/kg PO every 8 hours for otitis media

    Nursing drug reference: Dilute with 1 teaspoon (5 mL) of tap water and shake vigorously to yield 125 mg per 5 mL.

    The child weighs 25 kg.

    ▶ **How many milliliters will you give after reconstitution?** _____

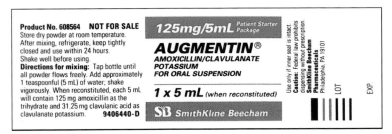

Courtesy of SmithKline Beecham Pharmaceuticals.

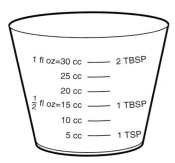

5. The physician orders heparin to infuse at 1300 units/hr continuous IV infusion.

    The pharmacy sends an IV bag labeled heparin 25,000 units in 250 mL.

    ▶ **Calculate the milliliters per hour to set the IV pump.** _____

6. A patient is receiving heparin 25,000 units in 250 mL infused at 25 mL/hr.

    ▶ **How many units per hour is the patient receiving?** _____

7. The physician orders morphine sulfate 2 mg/hr continuous IV for intractable pain related to end-stage lung cancer.

    The pharmacy sends an IV bag labeled morphine sulfate 100 mg in 250 mL.

    ▶ **Calculate the milliliters per hour to set the IV pump.** _____

8. Order: 1000 mL D5W/1/2 NS with 20 mEq of KCl to infuse in 12 hours

    Drop factor: 20 gtt/mL

    ▶ **Calculate the number of drops per minute.** _____

9. Order: Azactam 500 mg IV every 12 hours for septicemia

Supply: Azactam 1-g vials

Nursing drug reference: Dilute each 1-g vial with 10 mL of sterile water for injection and further dilute in 100 mL of NS to infuse over 60 minutes.

▶ **How many milliliters will you draw from the vial after reconstitution?** _____

▶ **Calculate the milliliters per hour to set the IV pump.** _____

▶ **Calculate the drops per minute with a drop factor of 20 gtt/mL.** _____

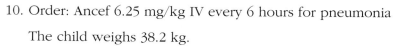

10. Order: Ancef 6.25 mg/kg IV every 6 hours for pneumonia

The child weighs 38.2 kg.

Nursing drug reference: Dilute each 1-g vial with 10 mL of sterile water for injection and further dilute 50 mL of NS to infuse over 30 minutes.

▶ **How many milliliters will you draw from the vial after reconstitution?** _____

▶ **Calculate the milliliters per hour to set the IV pump.** _____

▶ **Calculate the drops per minute with a drop factor of 10 gtt/mL.** _____

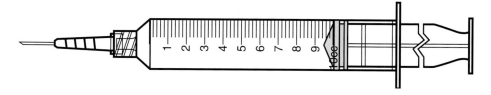

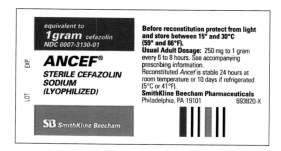

Courtesy of SmithKline Beecham Pharmaceuticals.

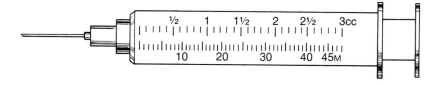

ANSWER KEY FOR CHAPTER 5: TWO-FACTOR MEDICATION PROBLEMS

Exercise 5.1 Pediatric Medication Problems Involving Weight

1. Sequential method:

$$\frac{1\ \cancel{mg}}{\cancel{kg}}\left|\frac{\cancel{mL}}{10\ \cancel{mg}}\right|\frac{1\ \cancel{kg}}{2.2\ \cancel{lb}}\left|\frac{45\ \cancel{lb}}{}\right|\frac{1\times1\times45}{10\times2.2}\left|\frac{45}{22}\right.=\frac{2.04\ \text{or}}{2\ \text{mL}}$$

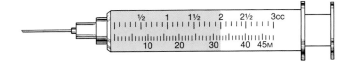

2. Sequential method:

$$\frac{0.01\ \cancel{mg}}{\cancel{kg}}\left|\frac{\cancel{mL}}{0.1\ \cancel{mg}}\right|\frac{1\cancel{kg}}{2.2\ \cancel{lb}}\left|\frac{20\ \cancel{lb}}{}\right|\frac{0.01\times1\times20}{0.1\times2.2}\left|\frac{0.2}{0.22}\right.=0.9\ \text{mL}$$

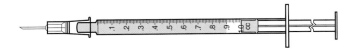

3. Sequential method:

$$\frac{0.5\ \cancel{mg}}{\cancel{kg}}\left|\frac{\cancel{mL}}{25\ \cancel{mg}}\right|\frac{1\ \cancel{kg}}{2.2\ \cancel{lb}}\left|\frac{45\ \cancel{lb}}{}\right|\frac{0.5\times1\times45}{25\times2.2}\left|\frac{22.5}{55}\right.=0.4\ \text{mL}$$

4. Random method:

$$\frac{5\theta\ \cancel{mcg}}{\cancel{kg}}\left|\frac{\cancel{mL}}{8\ \cancel{mg}}\right|\frac{1\ \cancel{mg}}{100\theta\ \cancel{mcg}}\left|\frac{1\ \cancel{kg}}{2.2\ \cancel{lb}}\right|\frac{75\ \cancel{lb}}{}\left|\frac{5\times1\times1\times75}{8\times100\times2.2}\right|\frac{375}{1760}=\text{mL}$$

$$\frac{375}{1760}=0.2\ \text{mL}$$

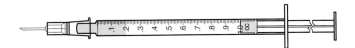

5. Random method:

$$\frac{10\ \cancel{mg}}{\cancel{kg}}\left|\frac{1\ \cancel{kg}}{2.2\ \cancel{lb}}\right|\frac{7\theta\ \cancel{lb}}{}\left|\frac{5\ \cancel{mL}}{300\ \cancel{mg}}\right|\frac{10\times1\times7\times5}{2.2\times30}\left|\frac{350}{66}\right.=5.3\ \text{or}\ 5\ \text{mL}$$

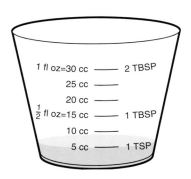

Exercise 5.2 Medication Problems Involving Reconstitution

1. Random method:

$$\frac{500\ \cancel{mg}}{\cancel{1\ g}}\left|\frac{50\ \cancel{mL}}{1000\ \cancel{mg}}\right|\frac{1\ \cancel{g}}{}\left|\frac{5\times5}{1}\right|\frac{25}{1}=25\ \text{mL}$$

2. Sequential method:

$$\frac{250\ \cancel{mg}}{500\ \cancel{mg}}\left|\frac{10\ \cancel{mL}}{}\right|\frac{25\times1}{5}\left|\frac{25}{5}\right.=5\ \text{mL}$$

3. Random method:

$$\frac{50\ \cancel{mg}}{\cancel{kg}}\left|\frac{4\ \cancel{mL}}{1.5\ \cancel{g}}\right|\frac{1\ \cancel{g}}{1000\ \cancel{mg}}\left|\frac{40\ \cancel{kg}}{}\right|\frac{5\times4\times1\times4}{1.5\times10}\left|\frac{80}{15}\right.=\frac{5.33\ \text{or}}{5\ \text{mL}}$$

Random method using yield:

$$\frac{50\ \cancel{mg}}{\cancel{kg}}\left|\frac{1\ \cancel{mL}}{375\ \cancel{mg}}\right|\frac{40\ \cancel{kg}}{}\left|\frac{50\times1\times40}{375}\right|\frac{2000}{375}=\frac{5.33\ \text{or}}{5\ \text{mL}}$$

4. Random method:

$$\frac{750\ \cancel{mg}}{\cancel{1\ g}}\left|\frac{20\ \cancel{mL}}{1000\ \cancel{mg}}\right|\frac{1\ \cancel{g}}{}\left|\frac{75\times2\times1}{1\times10}\right|\frac{150}{10}=15\ \text{mL}$$

5. Sequential method:

$$\frac{30 \text{ mg}}{\text{kg}} \left| \frac{5 \text{ (mL)}}{500 \text{ mg}} \right| \frac{1 \text{ kg}}{2.2 \text{ lb}} \left| \frac{65 \text{ lb}}{} \right| \frac{3 \times 5 \times 1 \times 65}{50 \times 2.2} \left| \frac{975}{110} \right| = \frac{8.86 \text{ or}}{8.9 \text{ mL}}$$

Exercise 5.3   Medication Problems Involving Intravenous Pumps

1. Sequential method:

$$\frac{1800 \text{ units}}{\text{(hr)}} \left| \frac{250 \text{ (mL)}}{25,000 \text{ units}} \right| \frac{18}{} = \frac{18 \text{ mL}}{\text{hr}}$$

2. Random method:

$$\frac{35 \text{ mg}}{\text{(hr)}} \left| \frac{250 \text{ (mL)}}{1 \text{ g}} \right| \frac{1 \text{ g}}{1000 \text{ mg}} \left| \frac{35 \times 25}{100} \right| \frac{875}{100} = \frac{8.75 \text{ or } 9 \text{ mL}}{\text{hr}}$$

3. Sequential method:

$$\frac{30 \text{ mL}}{\text{(hr)}} \left| \frac{25,000 \text{ (units)}}{250 \text{ mL}} \right| \frac{30 \times 2500}{25} \left| \frac{75,000}{25} \right| = \frac{3000 \text{ units}}{\text{hr}}$$

4. Sequential method:

$$\frac{15 \text{ mL}}{\text{(hr)}} \left| \frac{1 \text{ g}}{250 \text{ mL}} \right| \frac{1000 \text{ (mg)}}{1 \text{ g}} \left| \frac{15 \times 100}{25} \right| \frac{1500}{25} = \frac{60 \text{ mg}}{\text{hr}}$$

5. Sequential method:

$$\frac{900 \text{ units}}{\text{(hr)}} \left| \frac{500 \text{ (mL)}}{25,000 \text{ units}} \right| \frac{90 \times 5}{25} \left| \frac{450}{25} \right| = \frac{18 \text{ mL}}{\text{hr}}$$

Exercise 5.4   Medication Problems Involving Drop Factors

1. Sequential method:

$$\frac{800 \text{ mL}}{8 \text{ hr}} \left| \frac{15 \text{ (gtt)}}{\text{mL}} \right| \frac{1 \text{ hr}}{60 \text{ (min)}} \left| \frac{80 \times 15 \times 1}{8 \times 6} \right| \frac{1200}{48} = \frac{25 \text{ gtt}}{\text{min}}$$

2. Sequential method:

$$\frac{250 \text{ mL}}{} \left| \frac{15 \text{ gtt}}{\text{mL}} \right| \frac{\text{min}}{60 \text{ gtt}} \left| \frac{1 \text{ (hr)}}{60 \text{ min}} \right| \frac{250 \times 15 \times 1}{60 \times 60} \left| \frac{3750}{3600} \right| = \frac{1.04 \text{ or}}{1 \text{ hr}}$$

3. Sequential method:

$$\frac{150 \text{ mL}}{60 \text{ (min)}} \left| \frac{10 \text{ (gtt)}}{\text{mL}} \right| \frac{150 \times 1}{6} \left| \frac{150}{6} \right| = \frac{25}{6} \frac{\text{gtt}}{\text{min}}$$

4. Sequential method:

$$\frac{1000 \text{ mL}}{} \left| \frac{15 \text{ gtt}}{\text{mL}} \right| \frac{\text{min}}{50 \text{ gtt}} \left| \frac{1 \text{ (hr)}}{60 \text{ min}} \right| \frac{10 \times 15 \times 1}{5 \times 6} \left| \frac{150}{30} \right| = 5 \text{ hr}$$

5. Sequential method:

$$\frac{500 \text{ mL}}{4 \text{ hr}} \left| \frac{15 \text{ (gtt)}}{\text{mL}} \right| \frac{1 \text{ hr}}{60 \text{ (min)}} \left| \frac{50 \times 15 \times 1}{4 \times 6} \right| \frac{750}{24} = \frac{31.25 \text{ or } 31 \text{ gtt}}{\text{min}}$$

Exercise 5.5   Medication Problems Involving Intermittent Infusion

1. Random method:

$$\frac{250 \text{ mg}}{} \left| \frac{10 \text{ (mL)}}{1 \text{ g}} \right| \frac{1 \text{ g}}{1000 \text{ mg}} \left| \frac{25 \times 1}{10} \right| \frac{25}{10} = 2.5 \text{ mL}$$

Calculate milliliters per hour to set the IV pump. Sequential method:

$$\frac{52.5 \text{ (mL)}}{15 \text{ min}} \left| \frac{60 \text{ min}}{1 \text{ (hr)}} \right| \frac{52.5 \times 60}{15 \times 1} \left| \frac{3150}{15} \right| = \frac{210 \text{ mL}}{\text{hr}}$$

Calculate drops per minute with a drop factor of 10 gtt/mL. Sequential method:

$$\frac{52.5 \text{ mL}}{15 \text{ (min)}} \left| \frac{10 \text{ (gtt)}}{\text{mL}} \right| \frac{52.5 \times 10}{15} \left| \frac{525}{15} \right| = \frac{35}{\text{min}} \frac{\text{gtt}}{\text{min}}$$

2. Random method:

$$\frac{0.3 \text{ g}}{} \left| \frac{4 \text{ (mL)}}{600 \text{ mg}} \right| \frac{1000 \text{ mg}}{1 \text{ g}} \left| \frac{0.3 \times 4 \times 10}{6 \times 1} \right| \frac{12}{6} = 2 \text{ mL}$$

Calculate milliliter per hour to set the IV pump. Sequential method:

$$\frac{52 \text{ (mL)}}{15 \text{ min}} \left| \frac{60 \text{ min}}{1 \text{ (hr)}} \right| \frac{52 \times 60}{15 \times 1} \left| \frac{3120}{15} \right| = \frac{208 \text{ mL}}{\text{hr}}$$

Calculate drops per minute with a drop factor of 15 gtt/mL.
Sequential method:

$$\frac{52 \;\cancel{mL}}{15 \;\cancel{min}} \;\bigg|\; \frac{15 \;\text{(gtt)}}{\cancel{mL}} \;\bigg|\; \frac{52}{} = \frac{52}{} \;\frac{\text{gtt}}{\text{min}}$$

3. Sequential method:

$$\frac{3 \;\cancel{g}}{} \;\bigg|\; \frac{40 \;\text{(mL)}}{4 \;\cancel{g}} \;\bigg|\; \frac{3 \times 40}{4} \;\bigg|\; \frac{120}{4} = 30 \text{ mL}$$

Calculate milliliters per hour to set the IV pump.
Sequential method:

$$\frac{130 \;\text{(mL)}}{1 \;\text{(hr)}} \;\bigg|\; \frac{130}{1} = \frac{130}{} \;\frac{\text{mL}}{\text{hr}}$$

Calculate drops per minute with a drop factor of 20 gtt/mL.
Sequential method:

$$\frac{130 \;\cancel{mL}}{\cancel{1\,hr}} \;\bigg|\; \frac{20 \;\text{(gtt)}}{\cancel{mL}} \;\bigg|\; \frac{\cancel{1\,hr}}{60 \;\text{(min)}} \;\bigg|\; \frac{130 \times 2}{6} \;\bigg|\; \frac{260}{6} = 43.33 \text{ or } 43 \;\frac{\text{gtt}}{\text{min}}$$

4. Random method:

$$\frac{1000 \;\cancel{mg}}{} \;\bigg|\; \frac{4 \;\text{(mL)}}{1.5 \;\cancel{g}} \;\bigg|\; \frac{1 \;\cancel{g}}{1000 \;\cancel{mg}} \;\bigg|\; \frac{4 \times 1}{1.5} \;\bigg|\; \frac{4}{1.5} = \frac{2.66 \text{ or}}{2.7 \text{ mL}}$$

Calculate milliliters per hour to set the IV pump.
Sequential method:

$$\frac{102.7 \;\text{(mL)}}{1 \;\text{(hr)}} \;\bigg|\; \frac{102.7}{1} = \frac{102.7 \text{ or } 103}{} \;\frac{\text{mL}}{\text{hr}}$$

Calculate drops per minute with a drop factor of 20 gtt/mL.
Sequential method:

$$\frac{102.7 \;\cancel{mL}}{\cancel{1\,hr}} \;\bigg|\; \frac{20 \;\text{(gtt)}}{\cancel{mL}} \;\bigg|\; \frac{\cancel{1\,hr}}{60 \;\text{(min)}} \;\bigg|\; \frac{102.7 \times 2}{6} \;\bigg|\; \frac{205.4}{6} = 34.2 \text{ or } 34 \;\frac{\text{gtt}}{\text{min}}$$

5. Sequential method:

$$\frac{50 \;\cancel{mg}}{25 \;\cancel{mg}} \;\bigg|\; \frac{\text{(mL)}}{25} \;\bigg|\; \frac{50}{25} = 2 \text{ mL}$$

Calculate milliliters per hour to set the IV pump.
Random method:

$$\frac{52 \;\text{(mL)}}{30 \;\cancel{min}} \;\bigg|\; \frac{60 \;\cancel{min}}{1 \;\text{(hr)}} \;\bigg|\; \frac{52 \times 6}{3 \times 1} \;\bigg|\; \frac{312}{3} = 104 \;\frac{\text{mL}}{\text{hr}}$$

Calculate drops per minute with a drop factor of 10 gtt/mL.
Sequential method:

$$\frac{52 \;\cancel{mL}}{30 \;\text{(min)}} \;\bigg|\; \frac{10 \;\text{(gtt)}}{\cancel{mL}} \;\bigg|\; \frac{52 \times 1}{3} \;\bigg|\; \frac{52}{3} = 17.3 \text{ or } 17 \;\frac{\text{gtt}}{\text{min}}$$

Practice Problems

1. Sequential method:

$$\frac{0.2 \;\cancel{mg}}{\cancel{kg}} \;\bigg|\; \frac{2 \;\text{(mL)}}{5 \;\cancel{mg}} \;\bigg|\; \frac{1 \;\cancel{kg}}{2.2 \;\cancel{lb}} \;\bigg|\; \frac{10 \;\cancel{lb}}{} \;\bigg|\; \frac{0.2 \times 2 \times 1 \times 10}{5 \times 2.2} \;\bigg|\; \frac{4}{11} = \frac{0.36 \text{ or}}{0.4 \text{ mL}}$$

2. Sequential method:

$$\frac{10 \;\cancel{mg}}{\cancel{kg}} \;\bigg|\; \frac{5 \;\text{(mL)}}{160 \;\cancel{mg}} \;\bigg|\; \frac{8 \;\cancel{kg}}{} \;\bigg|\; \frac{1 \times 5 \times 8}{16} \;\bigg|\; \frac{40}{16} = 2.5 \text{ mL}$$

3. Sequential method:

$$\frac{1.25 \;\cancel{g}}{} \;\bigg|\; \frac{10 \;\text{(mL)}}{2 \;\cancel{g}} \;\bigg|\; \frac{1.25 \times 10}{2} \;\bigg|\; \frac{12.5}{2} = 6.25 \text{ or } 6.3 \text{ mL}$$

4. Random method:

$$\frac{750 \;\cancel{mg}}{} \;\bigg|\; \frac{4 \;\text{(mL)}}{1.5 \;\cancel{g}} \;\bigg|\; \frac{1 \;\cancel{g}}{1000 \;\cancel{mg}} \;\bigg|\; \frac{75 \times 4 \times 1}{1.5 \times 100} \;\bigg|\; \frac{300}{150} = 2 \text{ mL}$$

5. Sequential method:

$$\frac{700 \;\cancel{units}}{\text{(hr)}} \;\bigg|\; \frac{250 \;\text{(mL)}}{25,000 \;\cancel{units}} \;\bigg|\; \frac{7}{} = 7 \;\frac{\text{mL}}{\text{hr}}$$

6. Sequential method:

$$\frac{11 \text{ mL}}{\text{hr}} \left| \frac{15\theta \text{ mg}}{25\theta \text{ mL}} \right| \frac{11 \times 15}{25} \left| \frac{165}{25} \right. = 6.6 \frac{\text{mg}}{\text{hr}}$$

7. Sequential method:

$$\frac{1000 \text{ mL}}{8 \text{ hr}} \left| \frac{2\theta \text{ gtt}}{\text{mL}} \right| \frac{1 \text{ hr}}{6\theta \text{ min}} \left| \frac{1000 \times 2 \times 1}{8 \times 6} \right| \frac{2000}{48} = 41.66 \text{ or } 42 \frac{\text{gtt}}{\text{min}}$$

8. Sequential method:

$$\frac{75\theta \text{ mL}}{\text{mL}} \left| \frac{15 \text{ gtt}}{18 \text{ gtt}} \right| \frac{\text{min}}{6\theta \text{ min}} \left| \frac{1 \text{ hr}}{18 \times 6} \right| \frac{75 \times 15 \times 1}{18 \times 6} \left| \frac{1125}{108} \right. = \frac{10.41 \text{ or}}{10 \text{ hr}}$$

9. Sequential method:

$$\frac{1\theta \text{ mg}}{\text{kg}} \left| \frac{1\theta \text{ mL}}{5\theta\theta \text{ mg}} \right| \frac{1 \text{ kg}}{2.2 \text{ lb}} \left| \frac{20 \text{ lb}}{5 \times 2.2} \right| \frac{1 \times 1 \times 1 \times 20}{5 \times 2.2} \left| \frac{20}{11} \right. = 1.8 \text{ mL}$$

Sequential method:

$$\frac{101.8 \text{ mL}}{1 \text{ hr}} \left| \frac{101.8}{1} \right. = 101.8 \text{ or } 102 \frac{\text{mL}}{\text{hr}}$$

Sequential method:

$$\frac{101.8 \text{ mL}}{1 \text{ hr}} \left| \frac{1\theta \text{ gtt}}{\text{mL}} \right| \frac{1 \text{ hr}}{6\theta \text{ min}} \left| \frac{101.8 \times 1}{6} \right| \frac{101.8}{6} = 16.96 \text{ or } 17 \frac{\text{gtt}}{\text{min}}$$

10. Sequential method:

$$\frac{355 \text{ mg}}{} \left| \frac{1\theta \text{ mL}}{5\theta\theta \text{ mg}} \right| \frac{355 \times 1}{50} \left| \frac{355}{50} \right. = 7.1 \text{ or } 7 \text{ mL}$$

Calculate mL per hour to set the IV pump.

$$\frac{107 \text{ mL}}{1 \text{ hr}} \left| \frac{107}{1} \right. = 107 \frac{\text{mL}}{\text{hr}}$$

Calculate drops per minute with a drop factor of 20 gtt/mL.

Sequential method:

$$\frac{107 \text{ mL}}{1 \text{ hr}} \left| \frac{2\theta \text{ gtt}}{\text{mL}} \right| \frac{1 \text{ hr}}{6\theta \text{ min}} \left| \frac{107 \times 2}{6} \right| \frac{214}{6} = 35.66 \text{ or } 36 \frac{\text{gtt}}{\text{min}}$$

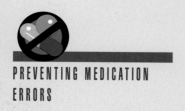

PREVENTING MEDICATION ERRORS

When medications are ordered for infants and children, the dosage of medication (g, mg, mcg, gr) based on the **weight** of the child must be considered as well as how much medication the child can receive per **dose** or **day.**

Although the **physician or nurse practitioner** orders the medications, the nurse must be aware of the safe dosage range for administration of medications. It is the responsibility of the nurse to check a nursing drug reference for the **right dosage** before administering a medication to a child to prevent **medication errors.**

When physicians or nurse practitioners order medications for critically ill patients, the patients must be closely monitored by the nurse for effectiveness of the medications. Often, the medications or intravenous (IV) fluids must be *titrated* for effectiveness, with an increase or decrease in the dosage based on the patient's response.

Factors involved in the safe administration of medications or IV fluids for the critically ill patient include the **dosage** of medication based on the **weight** of the patient and the **time** required for administration. The medication may need reconstitution or preparation by the nurse for immediate administration in a critical situation. The weight of the patient also may need to be obtained daily to ensure accurate correlation with the dosage of medication ordered. A nursing drug reference provides the nurse with information related to **dosage, weight,** and **time** for safe administration of medication.

To be able to calculate three-factor–given quantity to one-factor–, two-factor–, or three-factor–wanted quantity medication problems, it is necessary to understand all of the components of the medication order and to be able to calculate medication problems in a critical situation. This chapter will teach you to calculate medication problems involving the dosage of medication based on the weight of the patient and the time required for safe administration using dimensional analysis.

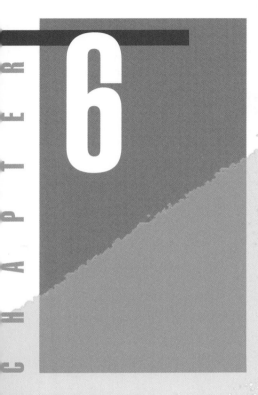

Outline

Exercise 6.1: Medication Problems Involving
Dosage, Weight, and Time   144
Practice Problems for Chapter 6:
Three-Factor Medication Problems   150
Post-Test for Chapter 6: Three-Factor
Medication Problems   153
Answer Key for Chapter 6:
Three-Factor Medication Problems   159

CHAPTER 6

Three-Factor Medication Problems

Objectives

After completing this chapter, you will be able to:

1. **Calculate three-factor–given quantity to one-factor–, two-factor–, or three-factor–wanted quantity medication problems involving a specific amount of medication or intravenous (IV) fluid based on the weight of the patient and the time required for safe administration.**
2. **Calculate problems requiring reconstitution or preparation of medications using information from a nursing drug reference, label, or package insert.**

Three-factor–given quantity medication problems can be solved implementing the sequential method or the random method of dimensional analysis. The *given quantity* or the physician's order now contains three parts, including a **numerator** (the *dosage* of medication ordered) and two **denominators** (the *weight* of the patient and the *time* required for safe administration).

Below is an example of this problem-solving method showing placement of basic dimensional analysis terms applied to a three-factor medication problem.

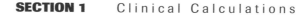

Unit Path

Given Quantity	Conversion Factor for Given Quantity (Numerator)	Conversion Factor for Given Quantity (Denominator)	Conversion Computation		Wanted Quantity
30 mg	5 mL	22 kg	$30 \times 5 \times 22$	3300	11 mL
kg/day	300 mg		300	= 300	day

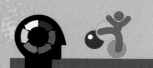

THINKING IT THROUGH

The three-factor–given quantity has been set up with a numerator (30 mg) and two denominators (kg/day) leading across the unit path to a two-factor–wanted quantity, with a numerator (mL) and a denominator (day). The conversion factors can now be factored into the unit path to allow cancellation of unwanted units.

The *dose on hand* (300 mg/5 mL) has been factored in and placed so that the wanted unit (mL) correlates with the *wanted quantity* (mL) and the unwanted unit (mg) is canceled.

The child's weight (22 kg) has been factored in and set up to allow the unwanted unit (kg) to be canceled.

All the unwanted units have been canceled, and the wanted units are placed to correlate with the two-factor–wanted quantity (mL/day). Multiply numerators, multiply denominators, and divide the product of the numerators by the product of the denom-

EXAMPLE 6.1

The physician orders Tagamet for gastrointestinal ulcers 30 mg/kg/day PO in four divided doses for a child weighing 22 kg. The dose on hand is Tagamet 300 mg/5 mL.

▶ **How many milliliters per day will the child receive?**

Given quantity = 30 mg/kg/day
Wanted quantity = mL/day
Dose on hand = 300 mg/5 mL
Weight = 22 kg

STEP 1 Identify the three-factor–given quantity (the physician's order), which contains three parts: a *numerator* (30 mg) and two denominators (kg/day). Establish the unit path from the given *quantity* (30 mg/kg/day) to the *two-factor–wanted quantity* (mL/day) using the sequential method of dimensional analysis and the necessary conversion factors.

Sequential method:

30 mg			mL
kg/day		=	day

STEP 2

Unit Path

Given Quantity	Conversion Factor for Given Quantity (Numerator)	Conversion Factor for Given Quantity (Denominator)	Conversion Computation		Wanted Quantity
30 ~~mg~~	5 (mL)				mL
kg/(day)	300 ~~mg~~			=	day

STEP 3

Unit Path

Given Quantity	Conversion Factor for Given Quantity (Numerator)	Conversion Factor for Given Quantity (Denominator)	Conversion Computation	Wanted Quantity
30 mg / kg/day	5 mL / 300 mg	22 kg		$= \dfrac{mL}{day}$

STEP 4

Unit Path

Given Quantity	Conversion Factor for Given Quantity (Numerator)	Conversion Factor for Given Quantity (Denominator)	Conversion Computation	Wanted Quantity
30 mg / kg/day	5 mL / 300 mg	22 kg	$\dfrac{3 \times 5 \times 22}{30} \quad \dfrac{330}{30}$	$= \dfrac{11\ mL}{day}$

STEP 5 Using dimensional analysis, calculate how many milliliters per dose the child should receive.

Given quantity = 11 mL/day
Wanted quantity = mL/dose

$$\dfrac{11\ mL}{day} = \dfrac{mL}{dose}$$

STEP 6

$$\dfrac{11\ mL}{day} \left| \dfrac{day}{4\ doses} \right| \dfrac{11}{4} = 2.75 \text{ or } \dfrac{2.8\ mL}{dose}$$

▶▶▶ *The wanted quantity is 2.8 mL/dose, and the child will receive this orally (PO) four times a day (qid).*

The problem could have been set up to find the wanted quantity of milliliters per dose.

STEP 6 (alternative).

Given quantity = 30 mg/kg/day
Wanted quantity = mL/dose
Dose on hand = 300 mg/5 mL
Weight = 22 kg

Sequential method:

$$\dfrac{30\ mg}{kg/day} \left| \dfrac{5\ mL}{300\ mg} \right| 22\ kg \left| \dfrac{day}{4\ doses} \right| \dfrac{3 \times 5 \times 22}{30 \times 4} \quad \dfrac{330}{120} = 2.75 \text{ or } \dfrac{2.8\ mL}{dose}$$

▶▶▶ *The wanted quantity is 2.8 mL/dose, and the child will receive this orally (PO) four times a day (qid).*

inators to provide the numerical answer. The wanted quantity is 11 mL/day.

The child is to receive 11 mL/day in four divided doses; therefore, the *conversion factor* involves how many doses are in a day (4 divided doses = day).

PREVENTING MEDICATION ERRORS

Every new medication order for a child should be carefully reviewed for errors related to **dosage, route,** and **frequency.** Many **medication errors** can be eliminated if a double-check system is in place for all new medication orders.

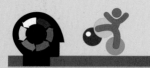

THINKING IT THROUGH

The *two-factor–given quantity* (2.8 mL/dose) has been factored in with a *numerator* (2.8 mL) and a *denominator* (dose). The *three-factor–wanted quantity* (mg/kg/day) also has been factored in with a *numerator* (mg) and two *denominators* (kg/day).

The *conversion factors* have been added, and all unwanted units have been canceled from the problem. The wanted unit (mg) is placed in the numerator to correlate with the *wanted quantity* (mg) also in the numerator. The wanted units (kg and day) are in the denominator to correlate with the wanted quantity (kg and day) in the denominator.

PREVENTING MEDICATION ERRORS

Knowing the **Five Rights** of medication administration can help to eliminate **medication errors** but another important consideration is being aware of the safe dosage range for each medication being administered.

A Nursing Drug Reference lists the safe dosage range for adults, children, and infants. It is the responsibility of the nurse to be familiar with safe dosage ranges to prevent **medication errors.**

EXAMPLE 6.2

As a prudent nurse, you are concerned that the child may be receiving an unsafe dosage of Tagamet; therefore, you want to identify how many milligrams per kilogram per day (mg/kg/day) the child weighing 22 kg is receiving. The dosage of medication being given four times a day is 2.8 mL/dose. The dosage on hand is 300 mg/5 mL.

▶ **How many milligrams per kilogram per day is the child receiving?**

Given quantity   = 2.8 mL/dose
Wanted quantity = mg/kg/dose
Dose on hand   = 300 mg/5 mL
Child's weight   = 22 kg

Sequential method:

STEP 1

$$\frac{2.8 \text{ mL}}{\text{dose}} \left| = \frac{\text{mg}}{\text{kg/day}}\right.$$

STEP 2

$$\frac{2.8 \text{ mL}}{\text{dose}} \left| \frac{300 \,\textcircled{mg}}{5 \text{ mL}} \right| \frac{4 \text{ doses}}{\textcircled{day}} \left| \frac{}{22 \,\textcircled{kg}} \right. = \frac{\text{mg}}{\text{kg/day}}$$

STEP 3

$$\frac{2.8 \,\cancel{\text{mL}}}{\cancel{\text{dose}}} \left| \frac{300 \,\textcircled{mg}}{5 \,\cancel{\text{mL}}} \right| \frac{\cancel{4 \text{ doses}}}{\cancel{\textcircled{day}}} \left| \frac{}{22 \,\textcircled{kg}} \right| \frac{2.8 \times 300 \times 4}{5 \times 22} \left| \frac{3360}{110} \right. = \frac{30.54 \text{ or } 30.5 \text{ mg}}{\text{kg/day}}$$

▶▶▶ *The three-factor–wanted quantity is 30.5 mg/kg/day. The nursing drug reference identifies that 20 to 40 mg/kg/day in four divided doses is a safe dosage of Tagamet for children. Therefore, the nurse is assured that the child is receiving a correct dosage. Dimensional analysis assists you to critically think through any type of medication problem.*

EXAMPLE 6.3

The physician orders dobutamine 5 mcg/kg/min IV for cardiac failure. The pharmacy sends an IV bag labeled: dobutamine 250 mg/50 mL D5W/0.45% NS. The patient weighs 165 lb.

▶ **Calculate the milliliters per hour at which to set the IV pump.**

Given quantity   = 5 mcg/kg/min
Wanted quantity = mL/hr
Dose on hand   = 250 mg/50 mL
Weight   = 165 lb

STEP 1 Identify the *three-factor–given quantity* (the physician's order) containing three parts, including the *numerator* (5 mg) and two *denominators* (kg/min). Establish the unit path from the three-factor–given quantity to the two-factor–wanted quantity (mL/hr).

Random method:

$$\frac{5 \text{ mcg}}{\text{kg/min}} = \frac{\text{mL}}{\text{hr}}$$

STEP 2

$$\frac{5 \text{ mcg}}{\text{kg/min}} \left| \frac{60 \text{ min}}{1 \text{ hr}} \right. = \frac{\text{mL}}{\text{hr}}$$

STEP 3

$$\frac{5 \text{ mcg}}{\text{kg/min}} \left| \frac{60 \text{ min}}{1 \text{ hr}} \right| \frac{50 \text{ mL}}{250 \text{ mg}} = \frac{\text{mL}}{\text{hr}}$$

STEP 4

$$\frac{5 \text{ mcg}}{\text{kg/min}} \left| \frac{60 \text{ min}}{1 \text{ hr}} \right| \frac{50 \text{ mL}}{250 \text{ mg}} \left| \frac{1 \text{ mg}}{1000 \text{ mcg}} \right. = \frac{\text{mL}}{\text{hr}}$$

STEP 5

$$\frac{5 \text{ mcg}}{\text{kg/min}} \left| \frac{60 \text{ min}}{1 \text{ hr}} \right| \frac{50 \text{ mL}}{250 \text{ mg}} \left| \frac{1 \text{ mg}}{1000 \text{ mcg}} \right| \frac{1 \text{ kg}}{2.2 \text{ lb}} \left| \frac{165 \text{ lb}}{} \right. = \frac{\text{mL}}{\text{hr}}$$

(Example continues on page 142)

THINKING IT THROUGH

The three-factor–given quantity has been set up with a *numerator* (5 mg) and *two denominators* (kg/min) leading across the unit path to a two-factor–wanted quantity with a *numerator* (mL) and a *denominator* (hr). By using the random method of dimensional analysis, the *conversion factors* are factored to cancel out unwanted units.

The unwanted unit (min) has been canceled by factoring the *conversion factor* (1 hr = 60 min), and the wanted unit corresponds with the *wanted quantity denominator* (hr).

The *dose on hand* (250 mg/50 mL) has been factored in and placed so that the *wanted unit* (mL) corresponds with the wanted quantity numerator (mL).

The *conversion factor* (1 mg = 1000 mcg) has been factored in to cancel the unwanted units (mg and mcg).

The final *conversion factors* (1 kg = 2.2 lb) and the *weight* of the patient have been factored in to cancel the remaining unwanted units (kg and lb). All the unwanted units have been canceled, and the wanted units (mL and hr) remain in position to correlate with the *two-factor–wanted quantity* (mL/hr). Multiply the numerators, multiply the denominators, and divide the product of the numerators by the product of the denominators to provide the numerical value for the two-factor–wanted quantity.

STEP 6

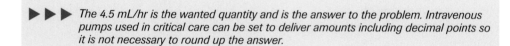

$$\frac{5 \text{ mcg}}{\text{kg/min}} \quad \frac{60 \text{ min}}{1 \text{ hr}} \quad \frac{50 \text{ mL}}{250 \text{ mg}} \quad \frac{1 \text{ mg}}{1000 \text{ mcg}} \quad \frac{1 \text{ kg}}{2.2 \text{ lb}} \quad \frac{165 \text{ lb}}{} = \frac{\text{mL}}{\text{hr}}$$

$$\frac{5 \times 6 \times 5 \times 1 \times 165}{25 \times 100 \times 2.2} \quad \frac{24,750}{5500} = \frac{4.5 \text{ mL}}{\text{hr}}$$

▶▶▶ *The 4.5 mL/hr is the wanted quantity and is the answer to the problem. Intravenous pumps used in critical care can be set to deliver amounts including decimal points so it is not necessary to round up the answer.*

THINKING IT THROUGH

The *two-factor–given quantity* is identified as the information that the nurse obtained from the IV pump, and the *three-factor–wanted quantity* is the information that the physician has requested.

The *dose on hand* (the IV fluid that is presently infusing) has been factored in to cancel the unwanted unit (mL).

The *conversion factor* (1 mg = 1000 mcg) has been factored in to cancel the unwanted unit (mg). The wanted unit (mcg) remains and corresponds with the wanted quantity in the *numerator*.

The *conversion factor* (1 hr = 60 min) has been factored in to cancel the unwanted unit (hr). The wanted unit (min) remains placed in the *denominator*.

The *conversion factor* (1 kg = 2.2 lb) has been factored in to correspond with the *wanted quantity denominator* (kg). The *weight* of the patient also is factored in to cancel the unwanted unit (lb). After all unwanted units have been canceled and the wanted units have been identi-

EXAMPLE 6.4

The nurse has been monitoring the hemodynamic readings of a patient weighing 165 lb receiving dobutamine, 250 mg in 50 mL of D5W/0.45% NS, and has received additional orders from the physician to *titrate* for effectiveness.

▶ **The IV pump is now set at 9 mL/hr, and the physician wants to know how many micrograms per kilogram per minute the patient is now receiving.**

Given quantity   = 9 mL/hr
Wanted quantity = mcg/kg/min
Dose on hand   = 250 mg/50 mL
Weight   = 165 lb

STEP 1

$$\frac{9 \text{ mL}}{\text{hr}} = \frac{\text{mcg}}{\text{kg/min}}$$

STEP 2

Sequential method:

$$\frac{9 \text{ mL}}{\text{hr}} \quad \frac{250 \text{ mg}}{50 \text{ mL}} = \frac{\text{mcg}}{\text{kg/min}}$$

STEP 3

$$\frac{9 \text{ mL}}{\text{hr}} \quad \frac{250 \text{ mg}}{50 \text{ mL}} \quad \frac{1000 \text{ mcg}}{1 \text{ mg}} = \frac{\text{mcg}}{\text{kg/min}}$$

fied, multiply the numerators, multiply the denominators, and divide the product of the numerators by the product of the denominators to provide the numerical value for the *wanted quantity.*

STEP 4

9 mL	250 mg	1000 mcg	1 hr		mcg
hr	50 mL	1 mg	60 min	=	kg/min

STEP 5

9 mL	250 mg	1000 mcg	1 hr	2.2 lb		mcg
hr	50 mL	1 mg	60 min	1 kg	165 lb	= kg/min

STEP 6

9 mL	250 mg	1000 mcg	1 hr	2.2 lb		mcg
hr	50 mL	1 mg	60 min	1 kg	165 lb	= kg/min

$$\frac{9 \times 25 \times 100 \times 2.2}{5 \times 6 \times 1 \times 165} \quad \frac{49,500}{4950} = \frac{10 \text{ mcg}}{\text{kg/min}}$$

▶▶▶ *The nurse can inform the physician that the patient is now receiving 10 mcg/kg/min infusing at 9 mL/hr.*

Dimensional analysis is a problem-solving method that uses critical thinking. When implementing the *sequential method* or the *random method* of dimensional analysis, the medication problem can be set up in a number of different ways, with a focus on the correct placement of *conversion factors* to allow unwanted units to be canceled from the unit path.

Dimensional analysis is a problem-solving method that nurses can use to calculate a variety of medication problems in the hospital, outpatient, or home care environment. The medication problems may involve one-factor–, two-factor–, or three-factor–given quantity medication orders, resulting in one-factor–, two-factor–, or three-factor–wanted quantity answers.

With advanced nursing and home care nursing resulting in increased autonomy, it is more important than ever that nurses be able to accurately calculate medication problems. Dimensional analysis provides the opportunity to use one problem-solving method for any type of medication problem, thereby increasing consistency and decreasing confusion when calculating medication problems.

PREVENTING MEDICATION ERRORS

When caring for critically ill patients, the nurse is responsible for titrating medication for the desired effectiveness (decrease in chest pain, increase in urine output, or increase in blood pressure).

The weight of a patient is extremely important when administering medications to a critically ill patient because a change in weight (either increased or decreased) can change the effectiveness of the medication. To prevent **medication errors,** a daily weight is obtained on every critically ill patient.

| **Exercise 6.1** | **Medication Problems Involving Dosage, Weight, and Time** |

(See page 159–160 for answers)

1. Order: furosemide 2 mg/kg/day PO in two divided doses for congestive heart failure

Supply: furosemide 40 mg/5 mL

Child's weight: 20 kg

▶ **How many milliliters per dose will you give?** _____

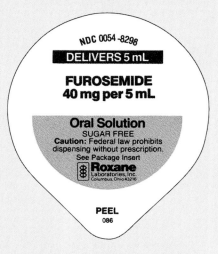

NDC 0054-8298

DELIVERS 5 mL

FUROSEMIDE
40 mg per 5 mL

Oral Solution
SUGAR FREE
Caution: Federal law prohibits
dispensing without prescription.
See Package Insert
Roxane
Laboratories, Inc.
Columbus, Ohio 43216

PEEL
086

Courtesy of Roxane Laboratories.

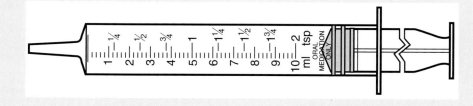

2. Order: Ancef 40 mg/kg/day in divided doses every 8 hours for infection

Supply: Ancef 1 g

Child's weight: 30 lb

Nursing drug reference: Reconstitute with 10 mL of sterile water for injection.

▶ **How many milliliters per dose will you draw from the vial after reconstitution?** _____

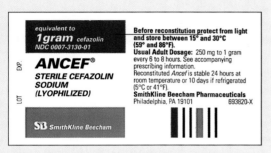

Courtesy of SmithKline Beecham Pharmaceuticals.

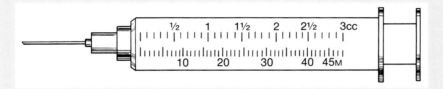

3. Order: Dilantin 6 mg/kg/day in divided doses every 12 hours for seizures

Supply: Dilantin 125 mg/5 mL

Child's weight: 45 lb

▶ **How many milliliters per dose will you give?** _____

(Exercise continues on page 146)

4. Order: prednisolone 1.5 mg/kg/day in four divided doses for inflammation

   Supply: prednisolone 6.7 mg/5 mL

   Child's weight: 20 kg

   ▶ **How many milliliters per dose will you give?** _____

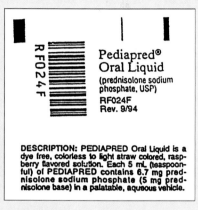

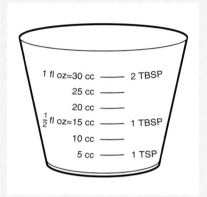

Courtesy of Fisons Pharmaceuticals.

5. Order: Cleocin 10 mg/kg/day IV in divided doses every 8 hours for infection

   Supply: Cleocin 300 mg/2 mL

   Child's weight: 50 lb

   ▶ **How many milliliters per dose will you give?** _____

Courtesy of Upjohn Company.

6. Order: dopamine 5 mcg/kg/min IV to increase blo...

Supply: dopamine 400-mg vial

Supply: 250 cc D5W

Patient's weight: 200 lb

▶ **How many milliliters will you draw from** ...
to equal 400 mg? _____

▶ **Calculate the milliliters per hour to set t** ...
IV pump. _____

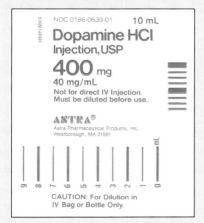

Courtesy of Astra Pharmaceutical
Products.

(Exercise continues on page 148)

Dopamine Hydrochloride Injection, USP

DOSAGE AND ADMINISTRATION
WARNING: This is a potent drug. It must be diluted before administration to patient.
Suggested Dilution
Transfer contents of one or more additive syringes of dopamine hydrochloride by aseptic technique to either a 250 mL, or 500 mL container of one of the following sterile intravenous solutions:

1. Sodium Chloride Injection, USP
2. Dextrose 5% Injection, USP
3. Dextrose (5%) and Sodium Chloride (0.9%) Injection, USP
4. Dextrose (5%) and Sodium Chloride (0.45%) Injection, USP
5. Dextrose (5%) in Lactated Ringer's Injection
6. Sodium Lactate (1/6 Molar) Injection, USP
7. Lactated Ringer's Injection, USP

Dopamine HCl has been found to be stable for a minimum of 24 hours after dilution in the sterile intravenous solutions listed above. However, as with all intravenous admixtures, dilution should be made just prior to administration.

Do NOT add dopamine HCl to 5% Sodium Bicarbonate or other alkaline intravenous solution, since the drug is inactivated in alkaline solution.

Rate of Administration
Dopamine HCl, after dilution, is administered intravenously through a suitable intravenous catheter or needle. An IV drip chamber or other suitable metering device is essential for controlling the rate of flow in drops/minute. Each patient must be individually titrated to the desired hemodynamic and/or renal response with dopamine HCl. In titrating to the desired increase in systolic blood pressure, the optimum dosage rate for renal response may be exceeded, thus necessitating a reduction in rate after the hemodynamic condition is stabilized.

Administration at rates greater than 50 mcg/kg/minute have safely been used in advanced circulatory decompensation states. If unnecessary fluid expansion is of concern, adjustment of drug concentration may be preferred over increasing the flow rate of a less concentrated dilution.

Suggested Regimen
1. When appropriate, increase blood volume with whole blood or plasma until central venous pressure is 10 to 15 cm H_2O or pulmonary wedge pressure is 14 to 18 mm Hg.
2. Begin administration of diluted solution at doses of 2–5 mcg/kg/minute dopamine HCl in patients who are likely to respond to modest increments of heart force and renal perfusion.

    In more seriously ill patients, begin administration of diluted solution at doses of 5 mcg/kg/minute dopamine HCl and increase gradually using 5–10 mcg/kg/minute increments up to 20–50 mcg/kg/minute as needed. If doses of dopamine HCl in excess of 50 mcg/kg/minute are required, it is suggested that urine output be checked frequently. Should urine flow begin to decrease in the absence of hypotension, reduction of dopamine HCl dosage should be considered. Multiclinic trials have shown that more than 50% of the patients were satisfactorily maintained on doses of dopamine HCl of less than 20 mcg/kg/minute. In patients who do not respond to these doses with adequate arterial pressures or urine flow, additional increments of dopamine HCl may be employed in an effort to produce an appropriate arterial pressure and central perfusion.
3. Treatment of all patients requires constant evaluation of therapy in terms of the blood volume, augmentation of myocardial contractility, and distribution of peripheral perfusion. Dosage of dopamine HCl should be adjusted according to the patient's response, with particular attention to diminution of established urine flow rate, increasing tachycardia or development of new dysrhythmias as indices for decreasing or temporarily suspending the dosage.
4. As with all potent administered drugs, care should be taken to control the rate of administration to avoid inadvertent administration of a bolus of drug.

Parenteral drug products should be inspected visually for particulate matter and discoloration prior to administration, whenever solution and container permit.

HOW SUPPLIED
Dopamine HCl 200 mg is supplied in the following form:
Additive Syringe   5 mL (40 mg/mL)   NDC 0186-0638-01

Dopamine HCl 800 mg is supplied in the following form:
Additive Syringe   5 mL (160 mg/mL) NDC 0186-0642-01

Dopamine HCl 400 mg is supplied in the following forms:
Additive Syringe   5 mL (80 mg/mL)   NDC 0186-0641-01
                    10 mL (40 mg/mL)   NDC 0186-0639-01

Packages are color coded according to the total dosage content; 200 mg coded blue/white, 400 mg coded green/white and 800 mg coded yellow/white.

Store at controlled room temperature 15°–30°C (59°–86°F). Protect from light.

Avoid contact with alkalies (including sodium bicarbonate), oxidizing agents, or iron salts.

NOTE: Do not use the Injection if it is darker than slightly yellow or discolored in any way.

ASTRA® | Astra Pharmaceutical Products, Inc.
Westborough, MA 01581

021861R07   3/92 (7)

Courtesy of Astra Pharmaceutical Products.

7. Information obtained by the nurse: Nipride 50 mg/250 mL D5W is infusing at 22 mL/hr.

    Patient's weight: 160 lb

    ▶ **How many micrograms per kilogram per minute is the patient receiving?** _____

8. Order: Inocor 5 mcg/kg/min IV for congestive heart failure

    Supply: Inocor 100 mg/100 mL of 0.9% NS

    Patient's weight: 180 lb

    ▶ **Calculate the milliliters per hour to set the IV pump.** _____

9. Information obtained by the nurse: Nipride 50 mg/250 mL D5W is infusing at 46 mL/hr.

   Patient's weight: 160 lb

   ▶ **How many micrograms per kilogram per minute is the patient receiving?** _____

10. Order: bretylium 5 mg/kg in 50 mL D5W IV over 30 minutes for arrhythmia

    Supply: bretylium 500-mg vial

    Patient's weight: 240 lb

    ▶ **How many milliliters will you draw from the vial to equal 500 mg?** _____

    ▶ **Calculate the milliliters per hour to set the IV pump.** _____

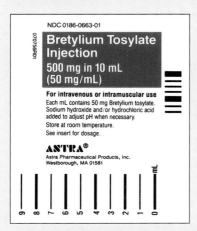

Courtesy of Astra Pharmaceutical Products.

Bretylium Tosylate Injection
For Intramuscular or Intravenous Use.

Suggested Bretylium Tosylate Admixture Dilutions and Administration Rates
for Continuous Infusion Maintenance Therapy Arranged in Descending Order of Concentration

PREPARATION				ADMINISTRATION		
Amount of Bretylium Tosylate	Volume of IV Fluid*	Final Volume	Final conc. (mg/mL)	Dose mg/min	Microdrops per min	mL/hour
FOR FLUID RESTRICTED PATIENTS: 500 mg (10 mL)	50 mL	60 mL	8.3	1.0 1.5 2.0	7 11 14	7 11 14
2 g (40 mL) 1 g (20 mL)	500 mL 250 mL	540 mL 270 mL	3.7 3.7	1.0 1.5 2.0	16 24 32	16 24 32
1 g (20 mL) 500 mg (10 mL)	500 mL 250 mL	520 mL 260 mL	1.9 1.9	1.0 1.5 2.0	32 47 63	32 47 63

*IV fluid may be either Dextrose Injection, USP or Sodium Chloride Injection, USP. This table does not consider the overfill volume present in the IV fluids.

Courtesy of Astra Pharmaceutical Products.

SUMMARY

This chapter has taught you to calculate three-factor medication problems involving the **dosage** of medication, the **weight** of the patient, and the amount of **time** over which medications or IV fluids can be safely administered. Using the sequential method or the random method of dimensional analysis, demonstrate your ability to calculate medication problems accurately by completing the following practice problems.

Practice Problems for Chapter 6	**Three-Factor Medication Problems**

(See pages 160–161 for answers)

1. Order: amrinone 8 mcg/kg/min IV for congestive heart failure

   Supply: amrinone 100 mg/100 mL of 0.9% NS

   Patient's weight: 198 lb

   ▶ **Calculate the milliliters per hour to set the IV pump.** _____

2. Order: Tagamet 40 mg/kg/day PO in four divided doses for gastro-

   intestinal ulcers

   Supply: Tagamet 300 mg/5 mL

   Child's weight: 80 lb

   ▶ **How many milliliters per dose will you give?** _____

3. Information obtained by the nurse: dopamine 200 mg in 500 mL D5W is

   infusing at 45 mL/hr for a patient weighing 60 kg.

   ▶ **How many micrograms per kilogram per minute is the patient receiving?** _____

4. Order: dopamine 2 mcg/kg/min IV for decreased cardiac output

   Supply: dopamine 400 mg/500 mL

   Patient's weight: 176 lb

   ▶ **Calculate the milliliters per hour to set the IV pump.** _____

5. Order: Neupogen 5 mcg/kg/day SQ for 2 weeks for neutropenia

   Supply: Neupogen 300 mcg/mL

   Patient's weight: 130 lb

   ▶ **How many micrograms per day will you give?** _____

6. Order: aminophylline 0.5 mg/kg/hr IV loading dose for bronchodilation

   Supply: aminophylline 250 mg/250 mL D5W

   Patient's weight: 132 lb

   ▶ **Calculate the milliliters per hour to set the
   IV pump.** _____

7. Order: furosemide 2 mg/kg/day PO for congestive heart failure

   Supply: furosemide 10 mg/mL

   Child's weight: 40 kg

   ▶ **How many milliliters per day will you give?** _____

8. Information obtained by the nurse: Nipride 200 mg in 1000 mL D5W is

   infusing at 15 mL/hr for a patient weighing 100 kg.

   ▶ **How many micrograms per kilogram per minute is the
   patient receiving?** _____

9. Information obtained by the nurse: A child weighing 65 lb is receiving

   10 mL of Tagamet PO qid from a stock bottle labeled: Tagamet

   300 mg/5 mL.

   ▶ **How many milligrams per kilogram per day is the
   child receiving?** _____

10. Information obtained by the nurse: aminophylline 250 mg/250 mL 0.9%

    NS is infusing at 25 mL/hr for a patient weighing 50 kg.

    ▶ **How many milligrams per kilogram per hour is the
    patient receiving?** _____

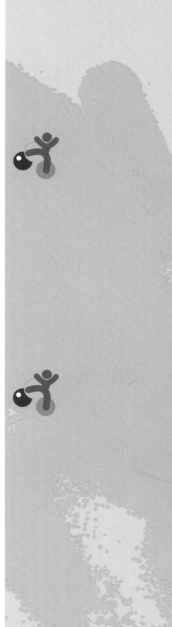

Chapter 6 Post-Test: Three-Factor Medication Problems

Name _____ **Date** _____

1. Order: morphine sulfate 0.3 mg/kg/dose PO every 4 hours for pain

   Supply: morphine sulfate 10 mg/5 mL

   Child's weight: 20 lb

   ▶ **How many milliliters per dose will you give?** _____

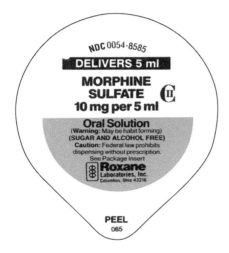

Courtesy of Roxane Laboratories, Inc.

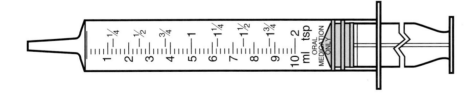

2. Order: filgrastim 5 mcg/kg/day for myelosuppression secondary to chemotherapy administration

   Supply: filgrastim 480 mcg/1.6 mL

   Patient's weight: 100 lb

   ▶ **How many milliliters per day will you give?** _____0.76_____

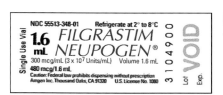

Courtesy of Amgen, Inc.

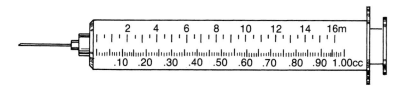

3. Order: Epogen 100 units/kg/day SQ three times weekly for anemia secondary to AZT administration

   Supply: Epogen 10,000 units/mL

   Patient's weight: 180 lb

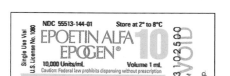

   ▶ **How many milliliters per day will you give?** _____

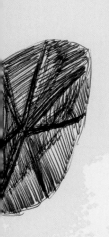

Courtesy of Amgen, Inc.

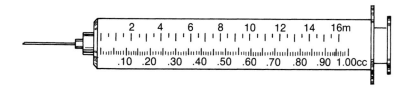

4. Order: digoxin 25 mcg/kg/day PO every 8 hours for congestive heart failure

Supply: digoxin 0.25 mg/5 mL

Child's weight: 25 lb

▶ **How many milliliters will you give per day?** _____5.7 ml / day_____

▶ **How many milliliters will you give per dose?** _____

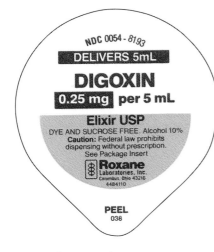

Courtesy of Roxane Laboratories, Inc.

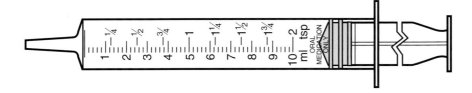

Handwritten annotations:

BID = 2x
TID = 3x

$$\frac{25\ mcg}{kg/day} \left| \frac{5\ ml}{0.25\ mg} \right| \frac{25\ lb}{2.2\ lb} \right| \frac{200 \times}{.25\ mg} \longrightarrow \frac{ml}{day}$$

1.9 ml/dose

5. Order: clindamycin 10 mg/kg/day IV in three divided doses for

   respiratory tract infection

   Supply: clindamycin 150 mg/mL

   Child's weight: 10 kg

   ▶ **How many milliliters per dose will you draw from the vial?** _0.22_

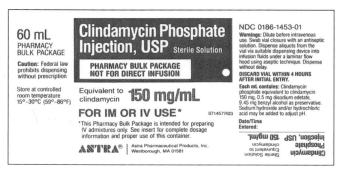

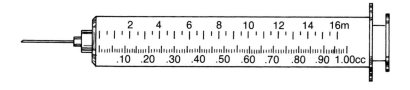

Courtesy of Astra Pharmaceutical Products.

6. Order: Claforan 100 mg/kg/day IV in two divided doses for infection

   Supply: Claforan 1 g/10 mL

   Neonate's weight: 2045 g

   ▶ **How many milliliters per dose will you draw from the vial?** _____

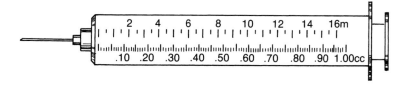

7. Order: gentamicin 2.5 mg/kg/dose IV every 12 hours for gram-negative

   bacillary infection

   Supply: gentamicin 40 mg/mL

   Neonate's weight: 1182 g

   ▶ **How many milligrams per dose will the neonate receive?** _____

8. Order: ampicillin 100 mg/kg/day IV in divided doses every 12 hours for respiratory tract infection

   Supply: ampicillin 125 mg/5 mL

   Neonate's weight: 1182 g

   ▶ **How many milligrams per dose will the neonate receive?** _____

   ▶ **How many milliliters per dose will you draw from the vial?** _____

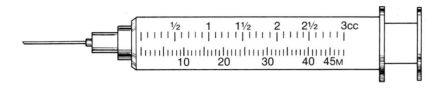

9. Order: Solu-Medrol 5.4 mg/kg/hr IV for acute spinal cord injury

   Supply: Solu-Medrol 125 mg/2 mL

   Patient's weight: 160 lb

   ▶ **How many milligrams per hour will the patient receive?** _____

10. Order: aminophylline 0.8 mg/kg/hr IV for respiratory distress

    Supply: aminophylline 250 mg/100 mL

    Child's weight: 65 lb

    ▶ **Calculate the milliliters per hour to set the IV pump.** _____

ANSWER KEY FOR CHAPTER 6: THREE-FACTOR MEDICATION PROBLEMS

Exercise 6.1 Medication Problems Involving Dosage, Weight, and Time

1. Sequential method:

$$\frac{2\ \text{mg}}{\text{kg/day}}\ \left|\ \frac{5\ \text{(mL)}}{40\ \text{mg}}\ \right|\ \frac{20\ \text{kg}}{}\ \left|\ \frac{\text{day}}{2\ \text{(doses)}}\ \right|\ \frac{2\times5\times2}{4\times2}\ \left|\ \frac{20}{8}\ \right.=2.5\ \frac{\text{mL}}{\text{dose}}$$

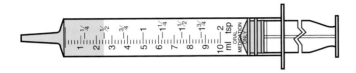

2. Random method:

$$\frac{40\ \text{mg}}{\text{kg/day}}\ \left|\ \frac{10\ \text{(mL)}}{1\ \text{g}}\ \right|\ \frac{\text{day}}{3\ \text{(doses)}}\ \left|\ \frac{1\ \text{kg}}{2.2\ \text{lb}}\ \right|\ \frac{30\ \text{lb}}{}\ \left|\ \frac{1\ \text{g}}{1000\ \text{mg}}\ \right.=\frac{\text{mL}}{\text{dose}}$$

$$\frac{4\times1\times3}{3\times2.2}\ \left|\ \frac{12}{6.6}\right.=1.81\ \text{or}\ 1.8\ \frac{\text{mL}}{\text{dose}}$$

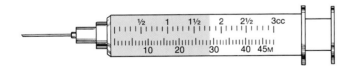

3. Sequential method:

$$\frac{6\ \text{mg}}{\text{kg/day}}\ \left|\ \frac{5\ \text{(mL)}}{125\ \text{mg}}\ \right|\ \frac{1\ \text{kg}}{2.2\ \text{lb}}\ \left|\ \frac{45\ \text{lb}}{}\ \right|\ \frac{\text{day}}{2\ \text{(doses)}}\ =\frac{\text{mL}}{\text{dose}}$$

$$\frac{6\times5\times1\times45}{125\times2.2\times2}\ \left|\ \frac{1350}{550}\right.=2.45\ \text{or}\ 2.5\ \frac{\text{mL}}{\text{dose}}$$

4. Sequential method:

$$\frac{1.5\ \text{mg}}{\text{kg/day}}\ \left|\ \frac{5\ \text{(mL)}}{6.7\ \text{mg}}\ \right|\ \frac{20\ \text{kg}}{}\ \left|\ \frac{\text{day}}{4\ \text{(doses)}}\ \right|\ \frac{1.5\times5\times20}{6.7\times4}\ =\frac{\text{mL}}{\text{dose}}$$

$$\frac{150}{26.8}=5.59\ \text{or}\ 5.6\ \frac{\text{mL}}{\text{dose}}$$

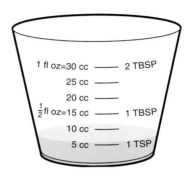

5. Sequential method:

$$\frac{10\ \text{mg}}{\text{kg/day}}\ \left|\ \frac{2\ \text{(mL)}}{300\ \text{mg}}\ \right|\ \frac{1\ \text{kg}}{2.2\ \text{lb}}\ \left|\ \frac{1\ \text{day}}{3\ \text{(doses)}}\ \right|\ \frac{50\ \text{lb}}{}\ \left|\ \frac{1\times2\times1\times1\times5}{3\times2.2\times3}\ \right|\ \frac{10}{19.8}=0.5\ \frac{\text{mL}}{\text{dose}}$$

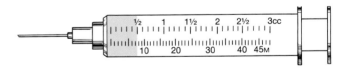

6. Sequential method:

$$\frac{400\ \text{mg}}{}\ \left|\ \frac{\text{(mL)}}{40\ \text{mg}}\ \right|\ \frac{40}{4}\ =10\ \text{mL}$$

Random method:

$$\frac{5\ \text{mcg}}{\text{kg/min}}\ \left|\ \frac{60\ \text{min}}{1\ \text{(hr)}}\ \right|\ \frac{1\ \text{kg}}{2.2\ \text{lb}}\ \left|\ \frac{200\ \text{lb}}{}\ \right|\ \frac{260\ \text{(mL)}}{400\ \text{mg}}\ \left|\ \frac{1\ \text{mg}}{1000\ \text{mcg}}\ \right.=\frac{\text{mL}}{\text{hr}}$$

$$\frac{5\times6\times2\times26\times1}{2.2\times4\times10}\ \left|\ \frac{1560}{88}\right.=17.7\ \text{or}\ 18\ \frac{\text{mL}}{\text{hr}}$$

7. Sequential method:

$$\frac{22\ \text{mL}}{\text{hr}}\left|\frac{50\ \text{mg}}{250\ \text{mL}}\right|\frac{1\ \text{hr}}{60\ \text{min}}\left|\frac{1000\ \text{mcg}}{1\ \text{mg}}\right|\frac{2.2\ \text{lb}}{1\ \text{kg}}\left|\frac{}{160\ \text{lb}}\right. = \frac{\text{mcg}}{\text{kg/min}}$$

$$\frac{22\times5\times10\times2.2}{25\times6\times1\times16}\left|\frac{2420}{2400}\right. = 1.008\ \text{or}\ 1\ \frac{\text{mcg}}{\text{kg/min}}$$

8. Random method:

$$\frac{5\ \text{mcg}}{\text{kg/min}}\left|\frac{100\ \text{mL}}{100\ \text{mg}}\right|\frac{1\ \text{mg}}{1000\ \text{mcg}}\left|\frac{1\ \text{kg}}{2.2\ \text{lb}}\right|\frac{180\ \text{lb}}{}\left|\frac{60\ \text{min}}{1\ \text{hr}}\right. = \frac{\text{mL}}{\text{hr}}$$

$$\frac{5\times1\times18\times6}{10\times2.2}\left|\frac{540}{22}\right. = 24.5\ \text{or}\ 25\ \frac{\text{mL}}{\text{hr}}$$

9. Sequential method:

$$\frac{46\ \text{mL}}{\text{hr}}\left|\frac{50\ \text{mg}}{250\ \text{mL}}\right|\frac{1\ \text{hr}}{60\ \text{min}}\left|\frac{1000\ \text{mcg}}{1\ \text{mg}}\right|\frac{2.2\ \text{lb}}{1\ \text{kg}}\left|\frac{}{160\ \text{lb}}\right. = \frac{\text{mcg}}{\text{kg/min}}$$

$$\frac{46\times5\times10\times2.2}{25\times6\times1\times16}\left|\frac{5060}{2400}\right. = 2.1\ \text{or}\ 2\ \frac{\text{mcg}}{\text{kg/min}}$$

10. Sequential method:

$$\frac{500\ \text{mg}}{}\left|\frac{\text{mL}}{50\ \text{mg}}\right|\frac{50}{5} = 10\ \text{mL}$$

Sequential method:

$$\frac{5\ \text{mg}}{\text{kg/30 min}}\left|\frac{60\ \text{mL}}{500\ \text{mg}}\right|\frac{1\ \text{kg}}{2.2\ \text{lb}}\left|\frac{240\ \text{lb}}{}\right|\frac{60\ \text{min}}{1\ \text{hr}} = \frac{\text{mL}}{\text{hr}}$$

$$\frac{5\times6\times24\times6}{3\times5\times2.2}\left|\frac{4320}{33}\right. = 130.9\ \text{or}\ 131\ \frac{\text{mL}}{\text{hr}}$$

Practice Problems

1. Random method:

$$\frac{8\ \text{mcg}}{\text{kg/min}}\left|\frac{100\ \text{mL}}{100\ \text{mg}}\right|\frac{1\ \text{mg}}{1000\ \text{mcg}}\left|\frac{1\ \text{kg}}{2.2\ \text{lb}}\right|\frac{198\ \text{lb}}{}\left|\frac{60\ \text{min}}{1\ \text{hr}}\right. = \frac{\text{mL}}{\text{hr}}$$

$$\frac{8\times1\times198\times6}{100\times2.2}\left|\frac{9504}{220}\right. = 43.2\ \frac{\text{mL}}{\text{hr}}$$

2. Sequential method:

$$\frac{40\ \text{mg}}{\text{kg/day}}\left|\frac{5\ \text{mL}}{300\ \text{mg}}\right|\frac{1\ \text{kg}}{2.2\ \text{lb}}\left|\frac{80\ \text{lb}}{}\right|\frac{\text{day}}{4\ \text{doses}} = \frac{\text{mL}}{\text{dose}}$$

$$\frac{4\times5\times1\times8}{3\times2.2\times4}\left|\frac{160}{26.4}\right. = 6.06\ \text{or}\ 6\ \frac{\text{mL}}{\text{dose}}$$

3. Sequential method:

$$\frac{45\ \text{mL}}{\text{hr}}\left|\frac{200\ \text{mg}}{500\ \text{mL}}\right|\frac{1000\ \text{mcg}}{1\ \text{mg}}\left|\frac{1\ \text{hr}}{60\ \text{min}}\right|\frac{}{60\ \text{kg}} = \frac{\text{mcg}}{\text{kg/min}}$$

$$\frac{45\times2\times10}{5\times6\times6}\left|\frac{900}{180}\right. = \frac{5\ \text{mcg}}{\text{kg/min}}$$

4. Random method:

$$\frac{2\ \text{mcg}}{\text{kg/min}}\left|\frac{500\ \text{mL}}{400\ \text{mg}}\right|\frac{1\ \text{mg}}{1000\ \text{mcg}}\left|\frac{60\ \text{min}}{1\ \text{hr}}\right|\frac{1\ \text{kg}}{2.2\ \text{lb}}\left|\frac{176\ \text{lb}}{}\right. = \frac{\text{mL}}{\text{hr}}$$

$$\frac{2\times5\times6\times1\times176}{4\times100\times2.2}\left|\frac{10{,}560}{880}\right. = \frac{12\ \text{mL}}{\text{hr}}$$

5. Random method:

$$\frac{5\ \text{mcg}}{\text{kg/day}}\left|\frac{1\ \text{kg}}{2.2\ \text{lb}}\right|\frac{130\ \text{lb}}{}\left|\frac{5\times1\times130}{2.2}\right|\frac{650}{2.2} = 295.45\ \text{or}\ 296\ \frac{\text{mcg}}{\text{day}}$$

6. Sequential method:

$$\frac{0.5 \text{ mg}}{\text{kg} / \text{hr}} \left| \frac{250 \text{ mL}}{250 \text{ mg}} \right| \frac{1 \text{ kg}}{2.2 \text{ lb}} \left| 132 \text{ lb} \right| \frac{0.5 \times 1 \times 132}{2.2} \left| \frac{66}{2.2} \right. = \frac{30 \text{ mL}}{\text{hr}}$$

7. Sequential method:

$$\frac{2 \text{ mg}}{\text{kg} / \text{day}} \left| \frac{\text{mL}}{10 \text{ mg}} \right| \frac{40 \text{ kg}}{} \left| \frac{2 \times 4}{1} \right| \frac{8}{1} = \frac{8 \text{ mL}}{\text{day}}$$

8. Sequential method:

$$\frac{15 \text{ mL}}{\text{hr}} \left| \frac{200 \text{ mg}}{1000 \text{ mL}} \right| \frac{1 \text{ hr}}{60 \text{ min}} \left| \frac{1000 \text{ mcg}}{1 \text{ mg}} \right| \frac{}{100 \text{ kg}} \left| \frac{15 \times 2}{60 \times 1} \right| \frac{30}{60} = \frac{0.5 \text{ mcg}}{\text{kg/min}}$$

9. Sequential method:

$$\frac{10 \text{ mL}}{\text{dose}} \left| \frac{300 \text{ mg}}{5 \text{ mL}} \right| \frac{4 \text{ doses}}{\text{day}} \left| \frac{2.2 \text{ lb}}{1 \text{ kg}} \right| \frac{}{65 \text{ lb}} = \frac{\text{mg}}{\text{kg/day}}$$

$$\frac{10 \times 300 \times 4 \times 2.2}{5 \times 1 \times 65} \left| \frac{26{,}400}{325} \right. = 81.23 \text{ or } 81 \frac{\text{mg}}{\text{kg/day}}$$

10. Sequential method:

$$\frac{25 \text{ mL}}{\text{hr}} \left| \frac{250 \text{ mg}}{250 \text{ mL}} \right| \frac{}{50 \text{ kg}} \left| \frac{25}{50} \right. = 0.5 \frac{\text{mg}}{\text{kg/hr}}$$

2

Practice Problems

Practice Problems | **One-Factor Practice Problems**
(See pages 199–202 for answers)

1. Order: Tigan 200 mg qid IM for nausea and vomiting

▶ **How many milliliters will you give?** _____

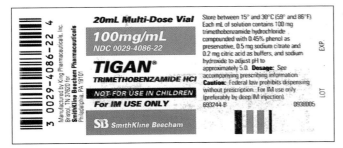

Courtesy of SmithKline Beecham Pharmaceuticals.

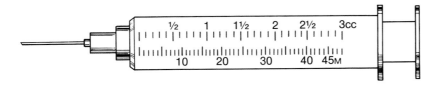

2. Order: morphine 30 mg PO every 4 hours for pain

▶ **How many tablets will you give?** _____

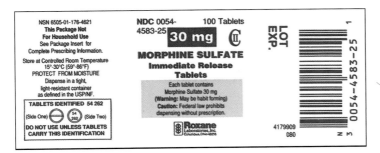

Courtesy of Roxane Laboratories.

(Practice Problems continue on page 166)

3. Order: prednisone 7.5 mg PO bid for inflammation

▶ **How many tablets will you give?** _____

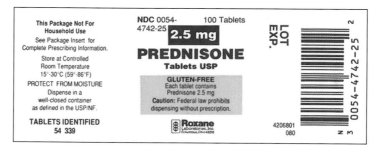

This Package Not For
Household Use

See Package Insert for
Complete Prescribing Information.

Store at Controlled
Room Temperature
15°-30°C (59°-86°F)

PROTECT FROM MOISTURE

Dispense in a
well-closed container
as defined in the USP/NF.

TABLETS IDENTIFIED
54 339

NDC 0054-4742-25   100 Tablets

2.5 mg

PREDNISONE
Tablets USP

GLUTEN-FREE
Each tablet contains
Prednisone 2.5 mg
Caution: Federal law prohibits
dispensing without prescription.

Roxane
Laboratories, Inc.
Columbus, Ohio 43216

4206801
080

LOT
EXP.

0054-4742-25

Courtesy of Roxane Laboratories.

4. Order: acetaminophen 160 mg PO every 4 hours for fever

▶ **How many teaspoons will you give?** _____

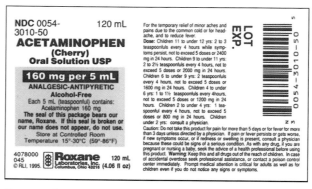

NDC 0054-3010-50   120 mL

ACETAMINOPHEN
(Cherry)
Oral Solution USP

160 mg per 5 mL
ANALGESIC-ANTIPYRETIC
Alcohol-Free
Each 5 mL (teaspoonful) contains:
Acetaminophen 160 mg
The seal of this package bears our
name, Roxane. If this seal is broken or
our name does not appear, do not use.
Store at Controlled Room
Temperature 15°-30°C (59°-86°F)

4078000
045
© RLI. 1995.

Roxane
Laboratories, Inc.
Columbus, Ohio 43216

120 mL
(4.06 fl oz)

For the temporary relief of minor aches and
pains due to the common cold or for headache, and to reduce fever.
Dose: Children 11 to under 12 yrs: 2 to 3
teaspoonfuls every 4 hours while symptoms persist, not to exceed 5 doses or 2400
mg in 24 hours. Children 9 under 11 yrs:
2 to 2½ teaspoonfuls every 4 hours, not to
exceed 5 doses or 2000 mg in 24 hours.
Children 6 to under 9 yrs: 2 teaspoonfuls
every 4 hours, not to exceed 5 doses or
1600 mg in 24 hours. Children 4 to under
6 yrs: 1 to 1½ teaspoonfuls every 4hours,
not to exceed 5 doses or 1200 mg in 24
hours. Children 2 to under 4 yrs: 1 teaspoonful every 4 hours, not to exceed 5
doses or 800 mg in 24 hours. Children
under 2 yrs: consult a physician.
Caution: Do not take this product for pain for more than 5 days or for fever for more
than 3 days unless directed by a physician. If pain or fever persists or gets worse,
if new symptoms occur, or if redness or swelling is present, consult a physician
because these could be signs of a serious condition. As with any drug, if you are
pregnant or nursing a baby, seek the advice of a health professional before using
this product. Warning: Keep this and all drugs out of the reach of children. In case
of accidental overdose seek professional assistance, or contact a poison control
center immediately. Prompt medical attention is critical for adults as well as for
children even if you do not notice any signs or symptoms.

LOT
EXP.

0054-3010-50

Courtesy of Roxane Laboratories.

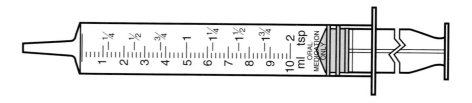

5. Order: Xanax 0.5 mg PO tid for anxiety

▶ **How many tablets will you give?** _____

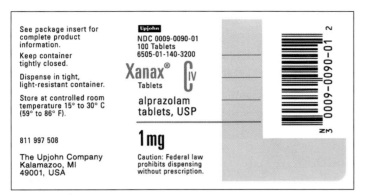

Courtesy of the Upjohn Company.

6. Order: Adalat 60 mg PO daily for hypertension

▶ **How many tablets will you give?** _____

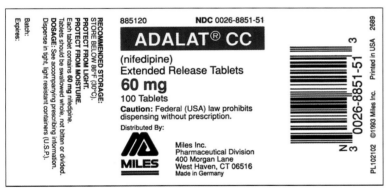

Courtesy of Miles Inc.

7. Order: Halcion 0.25 mg PO at hs for insomnia

▶ **How many tablets will you give?** _____

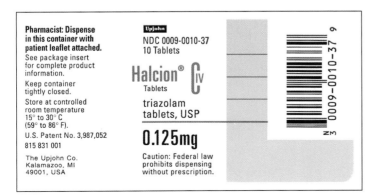

Courtesy of the Upjohn Company.

(Practice Problems continue on page 168)

8. Order: furosemide 80 mg PO daily for congestive heart failure

▶ **How many tablets will you give?** _____

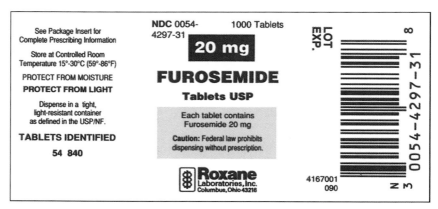

See Package Insert for
Complete Prescribing Information

Store at Controlled Room
Temperature 15°-30°C (59°-86°F)

PROTECT FROM MOISTURE
PROTECT FROM LIGHT

Dispense in a tight,
light-resistant container
as defined in the USP/NF.

TABLETS IDENTIFIED

54 840

NDC 0054-4297-31   1000 Tablets

20 mg

FUROSEMIDE

Tablets USP

Each tablet contains
Furosemide 20 mg

Caution: Federal law prohibits
dispensing without prescription.

Roxane
Laboratories, Inc.
Columbus, Ohio 43216

4167001
090

LOT
EXP.

3 0054-4297-31 8

Courtesy of Roxane Laboratories.

9. Order: morphine sulfate 10 mg IM prn for pain

▶ **How many milliliters will you give?** _____

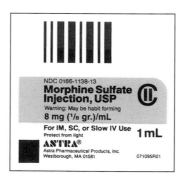

NDC 0186-1138-13
**Morphine Sulfate
Injection, USP**
Warning: May be habit forming
8 mg (⅛ gr.)/mL
For IM, SC, or Slow IV Use
Protect from light
ASTRA®
Astra Pharmaceutical Products, Inc.
Westborough, MA 01581   071095R01

1 mL

Courtesy of Astra Pharmaceutical Products.

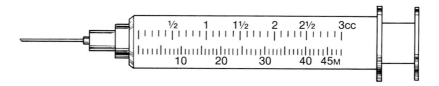

10. Order: naloxone HCl 100 mcg IVP prn for respiratory depression

▶ **How many milliliters will you give?** _____

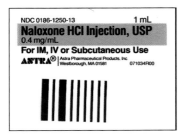

NDC 0186-1250-13   1 mL
Naloxone HCl Injection, USP
0.4 mg/mL
For IM, IV or Subcutaneous Use
ASTRA® | Astra Pharmaceutical Products, Inc.
Westborough, MA 01581   071034R00

Courtesy of Astra Pharmaceutical Products.

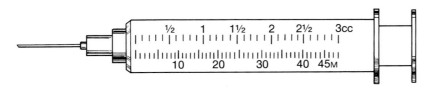

11. Order: Solu-Medrol 80 mg IVP every 4 hours for inflammation

▶ **How many milliliters will you give?** _____

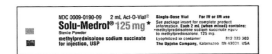

NDC 0009-0190-09   2 mL Act-O-Vial®   Single-Dose Vial   For IV or IM use
Solu-Medrol® 125 mg *   See package insert for complete product information. Each 2 mL (when mixed) contains:
Sterile Powder   •methylprednisolone sodium succinate equiv.
to methylprednisolone, 125 mg.
methylprednisolone sodium succinate   Lyophilized in container   812-393-303
for injection, USP   The Upjohn Company, Kalamazoo, MI 49001, USA

Courtesy of the Upjohn Company.

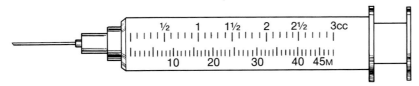

(Practice Problems continue on page 170)

12. Order: lactulose 20 g PO daily for constipation

▶ **How many milliliters will you give?** _____

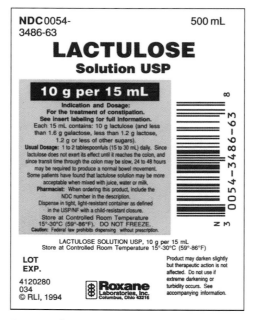

NDC 0054-3486-63   500 mL

LACTULOSE
Solution USP

10 g per 15 mL

Indication and Dosage:
For the treatment of constipation.
See insert labeling for full information.
Each 15 mL contains: 10 g lactulose (and less than 1.6 g galactose, less than 1.2 g lactose, 1.2 g or less of other sugars).
Usual Dosage: 1 to 2 tablespoonfuls (15 to 30 mL) daily. Since lactulose does not exert its effect until it reaches the colon, and since transit time through the colon may be slow, 24 to 48 hours may be required to produce a normal bowel movement. Some patients have found that lactulose solution may be more acceptable when mixed with juice, water or milk.
Pharmacist: When ordering this product, include the NDC number in the description.
Dispense in tight, light-resistant container as defined in the USP/NF with a child-resistant closure.
Store at Controlled Room Temperature 15°-30°C (59°-86°F). DO NOT FREEZE.
Caution: Federal law prohibits dispensing without prescription.

LACTULOSE SOLUTION USP, 10 g per 15 mL
Store at Controlled Room Temperature 15°-30°C (59°-86°F)

LOT
EXP.

4120280
034
© RLI, 1994

Roxane
Laboratories, Inc.
Columbus, Ohio 43216

Product may darken slightly but therapeutic action is not affected. Do not use if extreme darkening or turbidity occurs. See accompanying information.

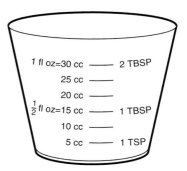

1 fl oz=30 cc —— 2 TBSP
25 cc ——
20 cc ——
½ fl oz=15 cc —— 1 TBSP
10 cc ——
5 cc —— 1 TSP

Courtesy of Roxane Laboratories.

13. Order: Compazine 5 mg IM tid for nausea and vomiting

▶ **How many milliliters will you give?** _____

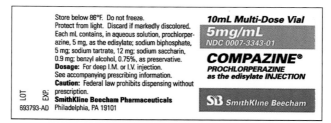

Store below 86°F. Do not freeze.
Protect from light. Discard if markedly discolored.
Each mL contains, in aqueous solution, prochlorperazine, 5 mg, as the edisylate; sodium biphosphate, 5 mg; sodium tartrate, 12 mg; sodium saccharin, 0.9 mg; benzyl alcohol, 0.75%, as preservative.
Dosage: For deep I.M. or I.V. injection.
See accompanying prescribing information.
Caution: Federal law prohibits dispensing without prescription.
SmithKline Beecham Pharmaceuticals
693793-AD   Philadelphia, PA 19101

LOT   EXP.

10mL Multi-Dose Vial
5mg/mL
NDC 0007-3343-01

COMPAZINE®
PROCHLORPERAZINE
as the edisylate INJECTION

SB SmithKline Beecham

Courtesy of SmithKline Beecham Pharmaceuticals.

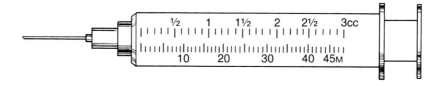

14. Order: Augmentin 250 mg PO every 8 hours for infection

▶ **How many milliliters will you give?** _____

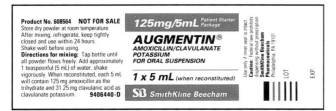

Courtesy of SmithKline Beecham Pharmaceuticals.

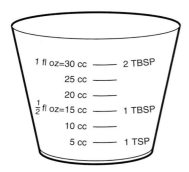

15. Order: Tigan 200 mg PO tid for nausea and vomiting

▶ **How many capsules will you give?** _____

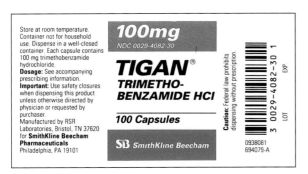

Courtesy of SmithKline Beecham Pharmaceuticals.

16. Order: prednisone 10 mg PO bid for adrenal insufficiency

▶ **How many tablets will you give?** _____

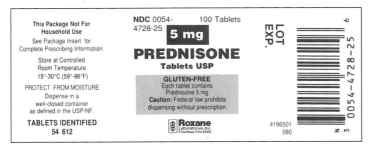

Courtesy of Roxane Laboratories.

(Practice Problems continue on page 172)

17. Order: hydromorphone 3 mg IM every 4 hours for pain

▶ **How many milliliters will you give?** _____

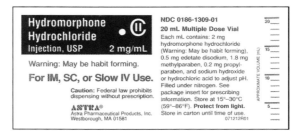

Courtesy of Astra Pharmaceutical Products.

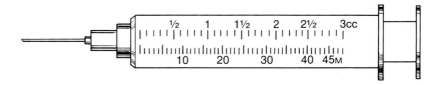

18. Order: acetaminophen 400 mg PO every 4 hours prn for fever

▶ **How many milliliters will you give?** _____

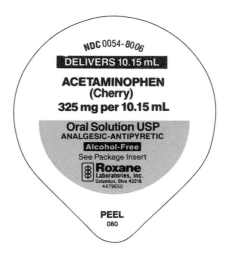

Courtesy of Roxane Laboratories.

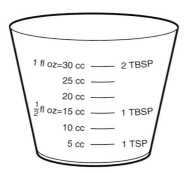

19. Order: magnesium sulfate 1000 mg IM times four doses for

hypomagnesemia

▶ **How many milliliters will you give?** _____

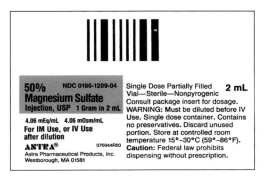

50% NDC 0186-1209-04
Magnesium Sulfate
Injection, USP 1 Gram in 2 mL

4.06 mEq/mL   4.06 mOsm/mL
For IM Use, or IV Use
after dilution
ASTRA®   070944R00
Astra Pharmaceutical Products, Inc.
Westborough, MA 01581

Single Dose Partially Filled   **2 mL**
Vial—Sterile—Nonpyrogenic
Consult package insert for dosage.
WARNING: Must be diluted before IV
Use. Single dose container. Contains
no preservatives. Discard unused
portion. Store at controlled room
temperature 15°–30°C (59°–86°F).
Caution: Federal law prohibits
dispensing without prescription.

Courtesy of Astra Pharmaceutical Products.

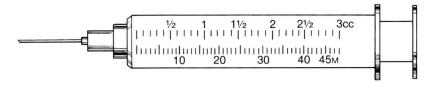

20. Order: Compazine 10 mg PO qid prn for nausea and vomiting

▶ **How many teaspoons will you give?** _____

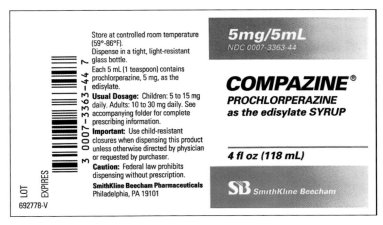

Store at controlled room temperature
(59°-86°F).
Dispense in a tight, light-resistant
glass bottle.
Each 5 mL (1 teaspoon) contains
prochlorperazine, 5 mg, as the
edisylate.
Usual Dosage: Children: 5 to 15 mg
daily. Adults: 10 to 30 mg daily. See
accompanying folder for complete
prescribing information.
Important: Use child-resistant
closures when dispensing this product
unless otherwise directed by physician
or requested by purchaser.
Caution: Federal law prohibits
dispensing without prescription.
SmithKline Beecham Pharmaceuticals
Philadelphia, PA 19101

5mg/5mL
NDC 0007-3363-44

COMPAZINE®
PROCHLORPERAZINE
as the edisylate SYRUP

4 fl oz (118 mL)

SB SmithKline Beecham

LOT EXPIRES
692778-V

Courtesy of SmithKline Beecham Pharmaceuticals.

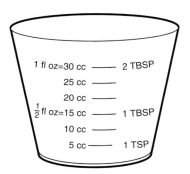

1 fl oz=30 cc ——— 2 TBSP
25 cc ———
20 cc ———
½ fl oz=15 cc ——— 1 TBSP
10 cc ———
5 cc ——— 1 TSP

(Practice Problems continue on page 174)

21. Order: Hemabate 0.25 mg IM to control postpartum bleeding

▶ **How many milliliters will you give?** _____

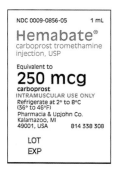

Courtesy of Pharmacia & Upjohn Company.

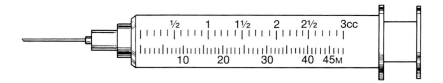

22. Order: Lincocin 500 mg every 8 hours IV for infection

▶ **How many milliliters will you draw from the vial?** _____

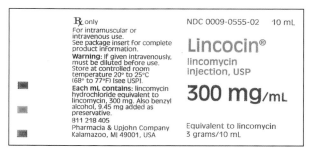

Courtesy of Pharmacia & Upjohn Company.

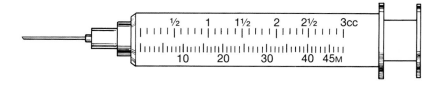

23. Order: Fragmin 2500 IU SQ daily for 10 days for thromboembolism prophylaxis

▶ **How many milliliters will you give?** _____

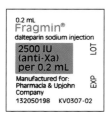

Courtesy of Pharmacia & Upjohn Company.

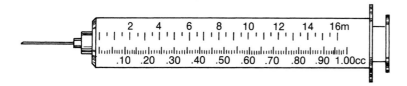

24. Order: Vantin 200 mg every 12 hours PO for infection

▶ **How many milliliters will you give?** _____

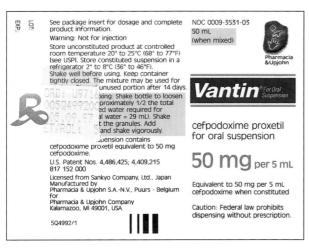

Courtesy of Pharmacia & Upjohn Company.

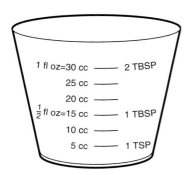

(Practice Problems continue on page 176)

25. Order: Cleocin 300 mg PO daily for *P. carinii* pneumonia

   ▶ **How many capsules will you give?** _____

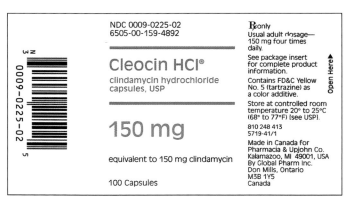

Courtesy of Pharmacia & Upjohn Company.

26. Order: Azulfidine 500 mg PO every 12 hours for management of

   inflammatory bowel disease

   ▶ **How many tablets will you give?** _____

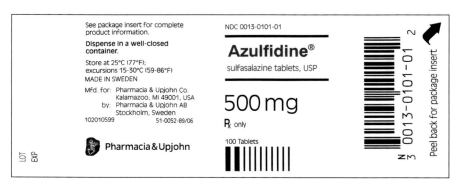

Courtesy of Pharmacia & Upjohn Company.

27. Order: Mirapex 0.25 mg PO tid for signs/symptoms of idiopathic

   Parkinson's disease

   ▶ **How many tablets will you give?** _____

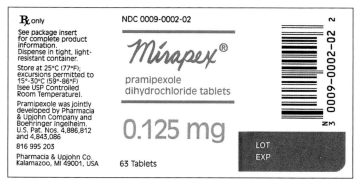

Courtesy of Pharmacia & Upjohn Company.

28. Order: Glyset 25 mg PO tid at the start of each meal for management of type 2 diabetes mellitus

▶ **How many tablets will you give?** _____

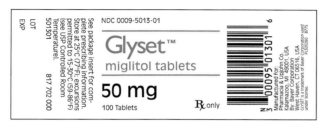

Courtesy of Pharmacia & Upjohn Company.

29. Order: Micronase 5 mg PO daily for control of blood sugars associated with non–insulin-dependent diabetes mellitus

▶ **How many tablets will you give?** _____

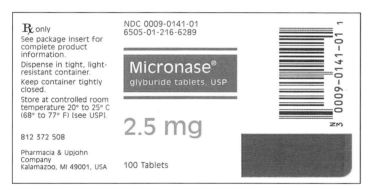

Courtesy of Pharmacia & Upjohn Company.

30. Order: Xanax 0.5 mg PO tid for panic attacks

▶ **How many tablets will you give?** _____

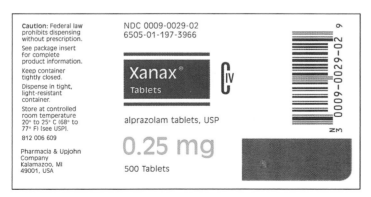

Courtesy of Pharmacia & Upjohn Company.

(Practice Problems continue on page 178)

31. Order: Depo-Provera 150 mg IM within the first 5 days of menses for contraception

▶ **How many milliliters will you give?** _____

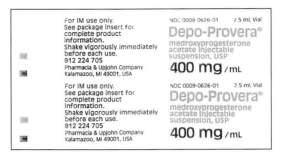

For IM use only.
See package insert for complete product information.
Shake vigorously immediately before each use.
812 224 705
Pharmacia & Upjohn Company
Kalamazoo, MI 49001, USA

NDC 0009-0626-01   2.5 mL Vial
Depo-Provera®
medroxyprogesterone acetate injectable suspension, USP
400 mg / mL

For IM use only.
See package insert for complete product information.
Shake vigorously immediately before each use.
812 224 705
Pharmacia & Upjohn Company
Kalamazoo, MI 49001, USA

NDC 0009-0626-01   2.5 mL Vial
Depo-Provera®
medroxyprogesterone acetate injectable suspension, USP
400 mg / mL

Courtesy of Pharmacia & Upjohn Company.

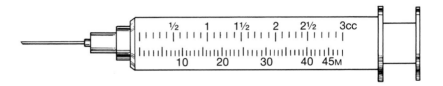

32. Order: Eskalith 600 mg PO tid initial dose followed by 300 mg PO qid for treatment of bipolar affective disorder. Check lithium levels every 3 months.

▶ **How many tablets will you give?** _____

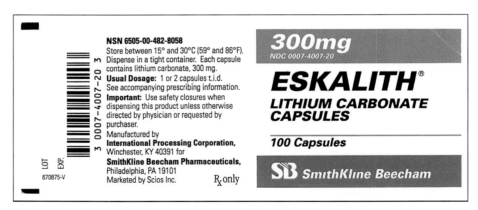

NSN 6505-00-482-8058
Store between 15° and 30°C (59° and 86°F).
Dispense in a tight container. Each capsule contains lithium carbonate, 300 mg.
Usual Dosage: 1 or 2 capsules t.i.d.
See accompanying prescribing information.
Important: Use safety closures when dispensing this product unless otherwise directed by physician or requested by purchaser.
Manufactured by
International Processing Corporation,
Winchester, KY 40391 for
SmithKline Beecham Pharmaceuticals,
Philadelphia, PA 19101
Marketed by Scios Inc.   Rₓonly
LOT
EXP.
670875-V

300mg
NDC 0007-4007-20
ESKALITH®
LITHIUM CARBONATE
CAPSULES
100 Capsules
SB SmithKline Beecham

Courtesy of SmithKline Beecham Pharmaceuticals.

Practice Problems | **Two-Factor Practice Problems**
(See pages 202–205 for answers)

1. Order: digoxin elixir 25 mcg/kg for congestive heart failure

   Child's weight: 25 lb

   ▶ **How many milliliters will you give?** _____

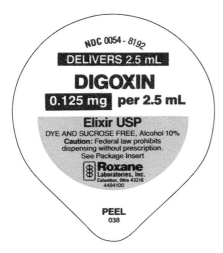

Courtesy of Roxane Laboratories.

2. Order: atropine sulfate 0.02 mg/kg IV every 4 hours for bradycardia

   Child's weight: 35 lb

   ▶ **How many milliliters will you give?** _____

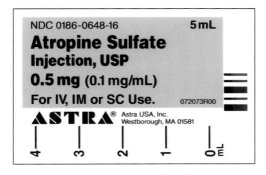

Courtesy of Astra Pharmaceutical Products.

(Practice Problems continue on page 180)

3. Order: lidocaine 2 mg/min IV for arrhythmia

   Supply: lidocaine 2 g/500 mL D5W

   ▶ **Calculate the milliliters per**
   hour to set the IV pump. _____

4. Order: Mezlin 1.5 g IV every 4 hours for infection

   Nursing drug reference: Reconstitute each 1 g with 10 mL of normal saline.

   ▶ **How many milliliters will you draw**
   from the vial alter reconstitution? _____

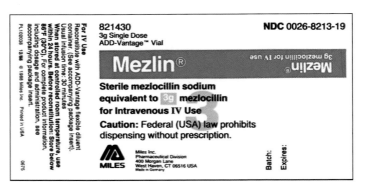

   Courtesy of Miles.

5. Order: gentamicin 1 mg/kg IV every 8 hours for infection

   Supply: gentamicin 40 mg/mL

   Child's weight: 94 lb

   ▶ **How many milliliters will you draw**
   from the vial? _____

6. Order: morphine 15 mg/hr IV for intractable pain

   Supply: morphine 300 mg/500 mL NS

   ▶ **Calculate the milliliters per**
   hour to set the IV pump. _____

7. Information obtained by the nurse: Dilaudid 50 mg in 250 mL NS is

   infusing at 25 mL/hr.

   ▶ **How many milligrams per hour**
   is the patient receiving? _____

8. Order: add 10 mEq KCl to 1000 mL D5W

   Supply: KCl 20 mEq/20 mL

   ▶ **How many milliliters will you draw
   from the vial to add to the IV bag?** _____

9. Information obtained by the nurse: nitroglycerin 50 mg in 500 mL D5W

   is infusing at 3 mL/hr.

   ▶ **How many micrograms per minute
   is the patient receiving?** _____

10. Information obtained by the nurse: 1000 mL D5W with 10 mEq KCl is

    infusing at 100 mL/hr.

    ▶ **How many milliequivalents of KCl
    is the patient receiving per hour?** _____

11. Order: infuse 1000 mL D5W at 250 mL/hr

    Drop factor: 20 gtt/mL

    ▶ **Calculate the number of drops
    per minute.** _____

12. Order: infuse 750 mL NS over 5 hours

    Drop factor: 10 gtt/mL

    ▶ **Calculate the number of drops
    per minute.** _____

13. Order: infuse 500 mL D5W over 8 hours

    Drop factor: 60 gtt/mL

    ▶ **Calculate the number of drops
    per minute.** _____

14. Order: infuse 750 mL D5W

    Drop factor: 15 gtt/mL

    Infusion rate: 18 gtt/min

    ▶ **Calculate the number of hours
    to infuse.** _____

(Practice Problems continue on page 182)

15. Order: infuse 250 mL NS

    Drop factor: 15 gtt/mL

    Infusion rate: 50 gtt/min

    ▶ **Calculate the number of hours to infuse.** _____

16. Order: infuse 1000 mL D5W/0.45% NS

    Drop factor: 15 gtt/mL

    Infusion rate: 25 gtt/min

    ▶ **Calculate the number of hours to infuse.** _____

17. Order: Fortaz 1.25 g IV every 12 hours for urinary tract infection

    Supply: Fortaz 2-g vial

    Nursing drug reference: Dilute each 1 g with 10 mL of sterile water and

    further dilute in 100 mL 0.9% NS to infuse over 1 hour.

    ▶ **How many milliliters will you draw from the vial after reconstitution?** _____

    ▶ **Calculate the milliliters per hour to set the IV pump.** _____

    ▶ **Calculate the drops per minute with a drop factor of 10 gtt/mL.** _____

18. Order: vancomycin 275 mg IV every 8 hours for infection

    Supply: vancomycin 500-mg vial

    Nursing drug reference: Reconstitute each 500-mg vial with 10 mL NS

    and further dilute with 250 mL NS to infuse over 1 hour.

    ▶ **How many milliliters will you draw from the vial after reconstitution?** _____

    ▶ **Calculate the milliliters per hour to set the IV pump.** _____

    ▶ **Calculate the drops per minute with a drop factor of 10 gtt/mL.** _____

19. Order: Mezlin 450 mg IV every 4 hours for infection

Supply: Mezlin 4-g vial

Nursing drug reference: Reconstitute each 1 g with 10 mL of sterile water and further dilute in 100 mL NS to infuse over 30 minutes.

▶ **How many milliliters will you draw from the vial after reconstitution?** _____

▶ **Calculate the milliliters per hour to set the IV pump.** _____

▶ **Calculate the drops per minute with a drop factor of 10 gtt/mL.** _____

20. Order: gentamicin 23 mg IV every 8 hours for infection

Supply: gentamicin 40 mg/mL

Nursing drug reference: Dilute with 100 mL NS and infuse over 1 hour.

▶ **How many milliliters will you draw from the vial after reconstitution?** _____

▶ **Calculate the milliliters per hour to set the IV pump.** _____

▶ **Calculate the drops per minute with a drop factor of 15 gtt/mL.** _____

(Practice Problems continue on page 184)

21. Order: Cortef 0.56 mg/kg PO daily for adrenal insufficiency

▶ **How many milliliters will you give a child weighing 18 kg?** _____

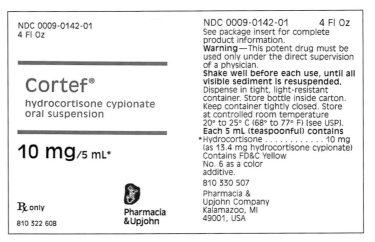

NDC 0009-0142-01
4 Fl Oz

Cortef®
hydrocortisone cypionate
oral suspension

10 mg/5 mL*

℞ only
810 322 608

Pharmacia
&Upjohn

NDC 0009-0142-01   4 Fl Oz
See package insert for complete
product information.
Warning—This potent drug must be
used only under the direct supervision
of a physician.
**Shake well before each use, until all
visible sediment is resuspended.**
Dispense in tight, light-resistant
container. Store bottle inside carton.
Keep container tightly closed. Store
at controlled room temperature
20° to 25° C (68° to 77° F) [see USP].
Each 5 mL (teaspoonful) contains
*Hydrocortisone . . . . 10 mg
(as 13.4 mg hydrocortisone cypionate)
Contains FD&C Yellow
No. 6 as a color
additive.
810 330 507
Pharmacia &
Upjohn Company
Kalamazoo, MI
49001, USA

Courtesy of Pharmacia & Upjohn Company.

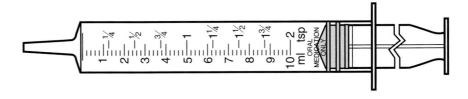

22. Order: Colestid 30 g/day PO in four divided doses for hyper-

cholesterolemia or management of cholesterol

▶ **How many packets/dose will you give?** _____

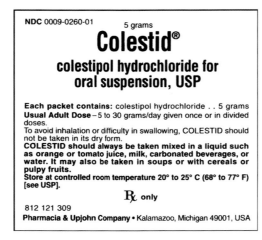

NDC 0009-0260-01   5 grams

Colestid®

**colestipol hydrochloride for
oral suspension, USP**

Each packet contains: colestipol hydrochloride . . 5 grams
Usual Adult Dose – 5 to 30 grams/day given once or in divided
doses.
To avoid inhalation or difficulty in swallowing, COLESTID should
not be taken in its dry form.
**COLESTID should always be taken mixed in a liquid such
as orange or tomato juice, milk, carbonated beverages, or
water. It may also be taken in soups or with cereals or
pulpy fruits.**
Store at controlled room temperature 20° to 25° C (68° to 77° F)
[see USP].

℞ only

812 121 309
Pharmacia & Upjohn Company • Kalamazoo, Michigan 49001, USA

Courtesy of Pharmacia & Upjohn Company.

23. Order: vincristine 10 mcg/kg IV weekly for treatment of Hodgkin's lymphoma

▶ **How many milliliters will you give a patient weighing 50 kg?** _____

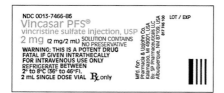

Courtesy of Pharmacia & Upjohn Company.

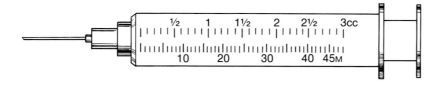

24. Order: Tagamet 1600 mg/day PO in two divided doses for gastro-esophageal reflux disease

▶ **How many tablets per dose will you give?** _____

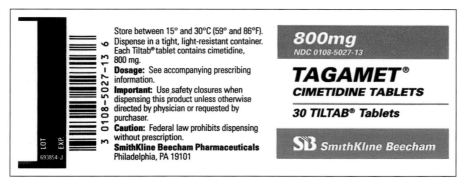

Courtesy of SmithKline Beecham Pharmaceuticals.

(Practice Problems continue on page 186)

25. Order: Thorazine 1 g/day PO in three divided doses for psychoses

▶ **How many milliliters per dose will you give?** _____

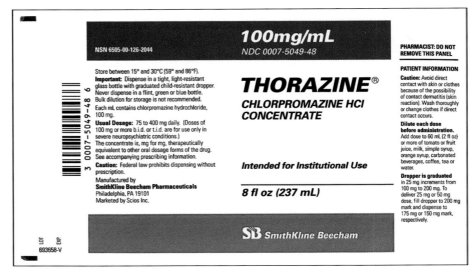

Courtesy of SmithKline Beecham Pharmaceuticals.

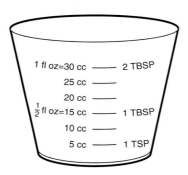

26. Order: Epivir 4 mg/kg PO bid for treatment of HIV infection

   ▶ **How many milliliters will you give a child weighing 20 kg?** _____

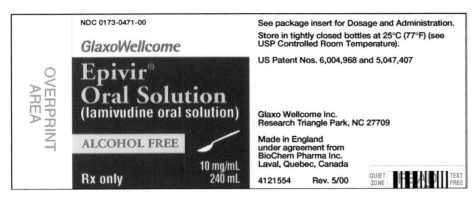

Courtesy of GlaxoWellcome.

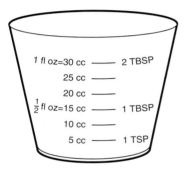

27. Order: Zofran 0.15 mg/kg IV 15 to 30 minutes before administration of chemotherapy for prevention of nausea and vomiting

   ▶ **How many milliliters will you give a patient weighing 160 lb?** _____

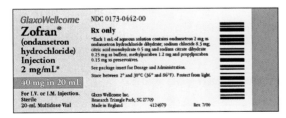

Courtesy of GlaxoWellcome.

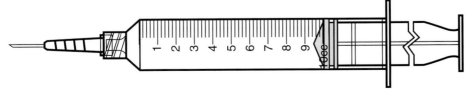

(Practice Problems continue on page 188)

28. Order: Epivir 2 mg/kg PO twice daily for treatment of HIV infection

    ▶ **How many tablets will you give a patient weighing 40 kg?** _____

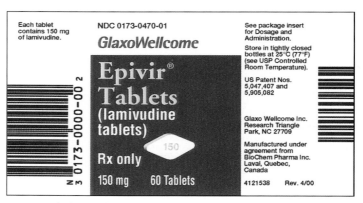

Courtesy of GlaxoWellcome.

29. Order: Zovirax 20 mg/kg PO qid for 5 days for treatment of chickenpox

    ▶ **How many tablets will you give a child weighing 20 lb?** _____

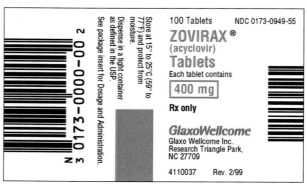

Courtesy of GlaxoWellcome.

30. Order: Wellbutrin SR 450 mg/day PO in three divided doses for treatment of depression

    ▶ **How many tablets per dose will you give?** _____

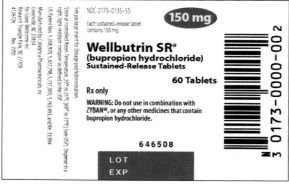

Courtesy of GlaxoWellcome.

31. Order: Zantac 2.4 g/day PO in four divided doses for treatment of duodenal ulcer

   ▶ **How many tablets per dose will you give?** _____

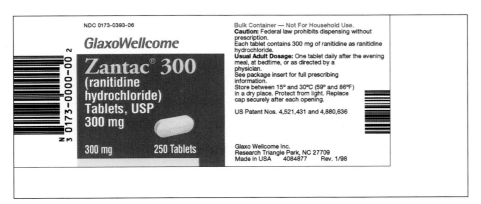

Courtesy of GlaxoWellcome.

32. Order: Zinacef 500 mg/day IV in two divided doses for urinary tract infection

   ▶ **How many milliliters per dose will you give?** _____

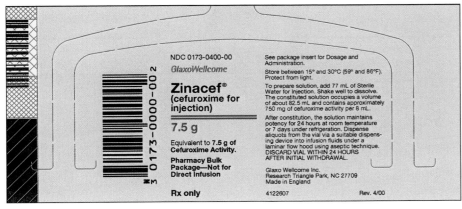

Courtesy of GlaxoWellcome.

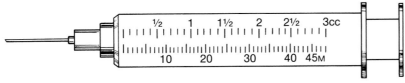

(Practice Problems continue on page 190)

33. Order: Ceptaz 1000 mg/day IV in two divided doses for treatment of respiratory tract infection

Nursing drug reference: Dilute each 1-g vial with 10 mL of normal saline.

▶ **How many milliliters per dose will you give?** _____

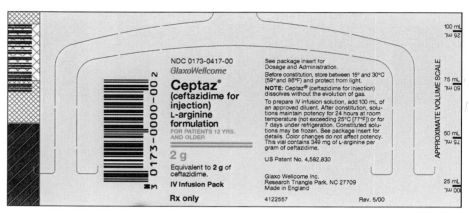

Courtesy of GlaxoWellcome.

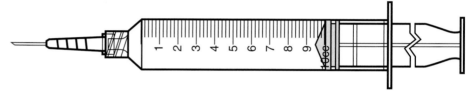

Practice Problems | **Three-Factor Practice Problems**
(See pages 205–207 for answers)

1. Order: Tagamet 40 mg/kg/day PO in four divided doses for treatment of active ulcer

Child's weight: 60 kg

▶ **How many milliliters per day will you give?** _____

▶ **How many milliliters per dose will you give?** _____

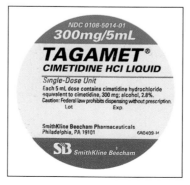

Courtesy of SmithKline Beecham Pharmaceuticals.

2. Order: furosemide 4 mg/kg/day IV for management of hypercalcemia of malignancy

Child's weight: 60 lb

▶ **How many milliliters per day will you give?** _____

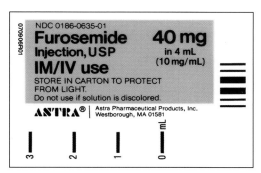

NDC 0186-0635-01

Furosemide   40 mg
Injection, USP   in 4 mL
IM/IV use   (10 mg/mL)

STORE IN CARTON TO PROTECT
FROM LIGHT.
Do not use if solution is discolored.

ASTRA® | Astra Pharmaceutical Products, Inc.
            | Westborough, MA 01581

Courtesy of Astra Pharmaceutical Products.

3. Order: Cleocin 30 mg/kg/day IV in divided doses every 8 hours for infection

Child's weight: 50 kg

▶ **How many milliliters per day will you give?** _____
▶ **How many milliliters per dose will you give?** _____

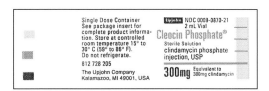

Single Dose Container
See package insert for
complete product informa-
tion. Store at controlled
room temperature 15° to
30° C (59° to 86° F).
Do not refrigerate.

812 728 205

The Upjohn Company
Kalamazoo, MI 49001, USA

Upjohn NDC 0009-0870-21
2 mL Vial
Cleocin Phosphate®
Sterile Solution
clindamycin phosphate
injection, USP

300mg Equivalent to
300mg clindamycin

Courtesy of the Upjohn Company.

4. Information obtained by the nurse: A child is receiving 0.575 mL/dose of gentamicin IV every 8 hours from a supply of gentamicin 40 mg/mL.

Child's weight: 45 lb

▶ **How many milligrams per kilogram per day
is the patient receiving?** _____

5. Information obtained by the nurse: A child is receiving 0.125 mL/dose of diphenhydramine (Benadryl) IV every 8 hours from a supply of Benadryl 50 mg/mL.

Child's weight: 20 lb

▶ **How many milligrams per kilogram per day
is the child receiving?** _____

(Practice Problems continue on page 192)

6. Order: dopamine 5 mcg/kg/min IV for decreased cardiac output

   Supply: dopamine 400-mg vial

   Nursing drug reference: Dilute each 400-mg vial in 250 mL NS

   Patient's weight: 110 lb

   ▶ **How many milliliters will you draw**
   from the vial? _____

   ▶ **Calculate the milliliters per hour to set**
   the IV pump. _____

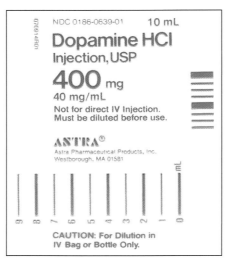

Courtesy of Astra Pharmaceutical Products.

7. Order: Nipride 0.8 mcg/kg/min IV for hypertensive crisis

   Supply: Nipride 50 mg/500 mL NS

   Patient's weight: 143 lb

   ▶ **Calculate the milliliters per hour to set**
   the IV pump. _____

8. Information obtained by the nurse: Nipride 50 mg in 250 mL NS is

   infusing at 68 mL/hr.

   Patient's weight: 250 lb

   ▶ **How many micrograms per kilogram**
   per minute is the patient receiving? _____

9. Order: Hydrea 30 mg/kg/day PO for ovarian carcinoma

   Patient's weight: 157 lb

   ▶ **How many grams per day is the**
   patient receiving? _____

10. Order: Venoglobulin-S 0.01 mL/kg/min for treatment of immuno-

   deficiency syndrome

   Patient's weight: 180 lb

   ▶ **Calculate the milliliters per hour to set
      the IV pump.** _____

11. Information obtained by the nurse: dopamine 400 mg in 250 mL D5W is

   infusing at 28 mL/hr.

   Patient's weight: 15 kg

   ▶ **How many micrograms per kilogram
      per minute is the patient receiving?** _____

12. Order: Inocor 3 mcg/kg/min IV for congestive heart failure

   Supply: Inocor 100 mg/100 mL of 0.9% NS

   Patient's weight: 160 lb

   ▶ **Calculate the milliliters per hour to set
      the IV pump.** _____

13. Order: Nipride 2 mcg/kg/min

   Supply: Nipride 50 mg/250 mL NS

   Patient's weight: 250 lb

   ▶ **Calculate the milliliters per hour to
      set the IV pump.** _____

14. Order: Nipride 1 mcg/kg/min IV for hypertensive crisis

   Supply: Nipride 50 mg/250 mL NS

   Patient's weight: 160 lb

   ▶ **Calculate the milliliters per hour to set
      the IV pump.** _____

15. Order: dopamine 2.5 mcg/kg/min IV for hypotension

   Supply: dopamine 400 mg/500 mL D5W

   Patient's weight: 65 kg

   ▶ **Calculate the milliliters per hour to set
      the IV pump.** _____

(Practice Problems continue on page 194)

16. Information obtained by the nurse: Isuprel 2 mg in 500 mL D5W is infusing at 15 mL/hr.

    Child's weight: 20 kg

    ▶ **How many micrograms per kilogram per minute is the child receiving?** _____

17. Order: Intropin 5 mcg/kg/min IV for treatment of oliguria after shock

    Supply: Intropin 400 mg/500 mL NS

    Patient's weight: 70 kg

    ▶ **Calculate the milliliters per minute.** _____

18. Order: vancomycin 40 mg/kg/day IV in three divided doses for infection

    Supply: vancomycin 500-mg vial

    Nursing drug reference: Reconstitute each 500-mg vial with 10 mL sterile water and further dilute in 100 mL of 0.9% NS to infuse over 60 minutes.

    Child's weight: 20 lb

    ▶ **How many milligrams per day is the child receiving?** _____

    ▶ **How many milligrams per dose is the child receiving?** _____

    ▶ **How many milliliters will you draw from the vial after reconstitution?** _____

    ▶ **Calculate the milliliters per hour to set the IV pump.** _____

19. Order: gentamicin 2 mg/kg/dose IV every 8 hours for infection

    Supply: gentamicin 40-mg/mL vial

    Nursing drug reference: Further dilute in 50 mL NS and infuse over 30 minutes.

    Child's weight: 40 kg

    ▶ **How many milligrams per dose is the child receiving?** _____

    ▶ **How many milliliters will you draw from the vial?** _____

    ▶ **Calculate the milliliters per hour to set the IV pump.** _____

20. Order: Ancef 25 mg/kg/day IV every 8 hours for infection

Supply: Ancef 500-mg vial

Nursing drug reference: Reconstitute each 500-mg vial with 10 mL of sterile water and further dilute in 50 mL NS to infuse over 30 minutes.

Child's weight: 25 kg

▶ **How many milligrams per day is the child receiving?** _____

▶ **How many milligrams per dose is the child receiving?** _____

▶ **How many milliliters will you draw from the vial after reconstitution?** _____

▶ **Calculate the milliliters per hour to set the IV pump.** _____

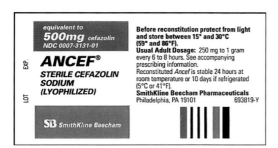

Courtesy of SmithKline Beecham Pharmaceuticals.

Practice Problems | **Comprehensive Practice Problems**
(See pages 208–209 for answers)

1. Order: digoxin 0.125 mg PO daily for congestive heart failure

On hand: digoxin 0.25 mg/tablet

▶ **How many tablets will you give?** _____

2. Order: ascorbic acid 0.5 g PO daily for supplemental therapy

On hand: ascorbic acid 500 mg/tablet

▶ **How many tablets will you give?** _____

3. Order: atropine gr 1/150 IM for on-call preanesthesia

Supply: atropine 0.4 mg/mL

▶ **How many milliliters will you give?** _____

(Practice Problems continue on page 196)

4. Order: Mycostatin oral suspension 500,000 units swish-and-swallow for oral thrush

   On hand: Mycostatin 100,000 units/mL

   ▶ **How many teaspoons will you give?** _____

5. Order: Demerol 50 mg IM every 4 hours for pain

   Supply: Demerol 100 mg/mL

   ▶ **How many milliliters will you give?** _____

6. Order: vancomycin 2 mg/kg IV every 12 hours for infection

   Supply: vancomycin 500 mg/10 mL

   Patient's weight: 75 kg

   ▶ **How many milliliters will you give?** _____

7. Order: ampicillin 2 mg/kg PO every 8 hours for infection

   Supply: ampicillin 500 mg/5 mL

   Patient's weight: 100 lb

   ▶ **How many milliliters will you give?** _____

8. Order: 1000 mL D5W to infuse in 12 hours

   Drop factor: 15 gtt/mL

   ▶ **Calculate the number of drops per minute.** _____

9. Order: 500 mL D5W

   Drop factor: 15 gtt/mL

   Infusion rate: 21 gtt/min

   ▶ **Calculate the hours to infuse.** _____

10. Order: heparin 1500 units/hr

    Supply: 250-mL IV bag of D5W with 25,000 units of heparin

    ▶ **Calculate the milliliters per hour to set the IV pump.** _____

11. Order: 1000 mL NS IV

    Drop factor: 15 gtt/mL

    Infusion rate: 50 gtt/min

    ▶ **Calculate the hours to infuse.** _____

12. Order: regular insulin 8 units per hour IV for hyperglycemia

    Supply: 250 mL NS with 100 units of regular insulin

    ▶ **Calculate the milliliters per hour to set the IV pump.** _____

13. Order: 500 mL of 10% lipids to infuse in 8 hours

    Drop factor: 10 gtt/mL

    ▶ **Calculate the number of drops per minute.** _____

14. Order: KCl 2 mEq/100 mL of D5W for hypokalemia

    On hand: 20 mEq/10-mL vial

    Supply: 500 mL D5W

    ▶ **How many milliliters of KCl will you add to the IV bag?** _____

15. Order: aminophylline 44 mg/hr IV for bronchodilation

    Supply: 250 mL D5W with 1 g of aminophylline

    ▶ **Calculate the milliliters per hour to set the IV pump.** _____

16. Order: Dilaudid 140 mL/hr

    Supply: 1000 mL D5W/NS with 30 mg of Dilaudid

    ▶ **Calculate the milligrams per hour that the patient is receiving.** _____

17. Order: Staphcillin 750 mg IV every 4 hours for infection

    Supply: Staphcillin 6 g

    Nursing drug reference: Reconstitute with 8.6 mL of sterile water to yield

    500 mg/mL and further dilute in 100 mL of NS to infuse over 30 minutes.

    ▶ **How many milliliters will you draw from the vial after reconstitution?** _____

    ▶ **Calculate the milliliters per hour to set the IV pump.** _____

    ▶ **Calculate the drops per minute with a drop factor of 10 gtt/mL.** _____

(Practice Problems continue on page 198)

18. Order: Pipracil 1.5 g every 6 hours for uncomplicated urinary

    tract infection

    Supply: Pipracil 3-g vial

    Nursing drug reference: Reconstitute each 3-g vial with 5 mL of sterile

    water and further dilute in 50 mL of 0.9% NS to infuse over 20 minutes.

    ▶ **How many milliliters will you draw from the
      vial after reconstitution?** _____

    ▶ **Calculate the milliliters per hour
      to set the IV pump.** _____

    ▶ **Calculate the drops per minute with
      a drop factor of 20 gtt/mL.** _____

19. Order: dopamine 4 mcg/kg/min IV for decreased cardiac output

    Supply: 250 mL D5W with 400 mg of dopamine

    Patient's weight: 120 lb

    ▶ **Calculate the milliliters per hour
      to set the IV pump.** _____

20. Order: Nipride 0.8 mcg/kg/min IV for hypertension

    Supply: 500 mL D5W with 50 mg Nipride

    Patient's weight: 143 lb

    ▶ **Calculate the milliliters per hour
      to set the IV pump.** _____

ANSWER KEY FOR SECTION 2: PRACTICE PROBLEMS

One-Factor Practice Problems

1. Sequential method:

$$\frac{200\ \text{mg}}{} \left|\ \frac{\text{mL}}{100\ \text{mg}}\ \right|\ \frac{2}{1} = 2\ \text{mL}$$

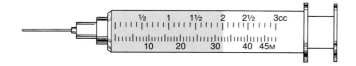

2. Sequential method:

$$\frac{30\ \text{mg}}{} \left|\ \frac{\text{tablet}}{30\ \text{mg}}\ \right|\ \frac{3}{3} = 1\ \text{tablet}$$

3. Sequential method:

$$\frac{7.5\ \text{mg}}{} \left|\ \frac{\text{tablet}}{2.5\ \text{mg}}\ \right|\ \frac{7.5}{2.5} = 3\ \text{tablets}$$

4. Sequential method:

$$\frac{160\ \text{mg}}{} \left|\ \frac{5\ \text{mL}}{160\ \text{mg}}\ \right|\ \frac{1\ \text{tsp}}{5\ \text{mL}}\ \right|\ \frac{1}{} = 1\ \text{tsp}$$

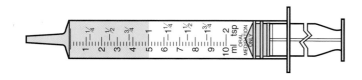

5. Sequential method:

$$\frac{0.5\ \text{mg}}{} \left|\ \frac{\text{tablet}}{1\ \text{mg}}\ \right|\ \frac{0.5}{1} = 0.5\ \text{tablet}$$

6. Sequential method:

$$\frac{60\ \text{mg}}{} \left|\ \frac{\text{tablet}}{60\ \text{mg}}\ \right| = 1\ \text{tablet}$$

7. Sequential method:

$$\frac{0.25\ \text{mg}}{} \left|\ \frac{\text{tablet}}{0.125\ \text{mg}}\ \right|\ \frac{0.25}{0.125} = 2\ \text{tablets}$$

8. Sequential method:

$$\frac{80\ \text{mg}}{} \left|\ \frac{\text{tablet}}{20\ \text{mg}}\ \right|\ \frac{8}{2} = 4\ \text{tablets}$$

9. Random method:

$$\frac{10\ \text{mg}}{} \left|\ \frac{\text{mL}}{\frac{1}{8}\text{gr}}\ \right|\ \frac{1\ \text{gr}}{60\ \text{mg}}\ \right|\ \frac{1 \times 1}{\frac{1}{8} \times \frac{6}{1}}\ \right|\ \frac{1}{\frac{6}{8}}\ \right|\ \frac{1}{0.75} = \begin{array}{l}1.33\ \text{or}\\ 1.3\ \text{mL}\end{array}$$

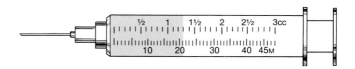

10. Random method:

$$\frac{100\ \text{mcg}}{} \left|\ \frac{\text{mL}}{0.4\ \text{mg}}\ \right|\ \frac{1\ \text{mg}}{1000\ \text{mcg}}\ \right|\ \frac{1 \times 1}{0.4 \times 10}\ \right|\ \frac{1}{4} = \begin{array}{l}0.25\ \text{or}\\ 0.3\ \text{mL}\end{array}$$

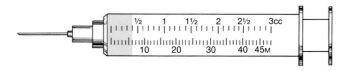

11. Sequential method:

$$\frac{80\ \text{mg}}{} \left|\ \frac{2\ \text{mL}}{125\ \text{mg}}\ \right|\ \frac{80 \times 2}{125}\ \right|\ \frac{160}{125} = 1.28\ \text{or}\ 1.3\ \text{mL}$$

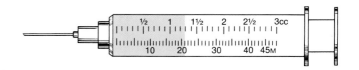

12. Sequential method:

$$\frac{20\ \cancel{g}\ |\ 15\ \boxed{mL}\ |\ 2\times15\ |\ 30}{|\ 10\ \cancel{g}\ |\ 1\ |\ 1} = 30\ mL$$

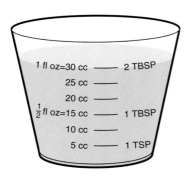

13. Sequential method:

$$\frac{\cancel{5\ mg}\ |\ \boxed{mL}}{|\ \cancel{5\ mg}} = 1\ mL$$

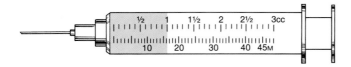

14. Sequential method:

$$\frac{250\ \cancel{mg}\ |\ 5\ \boxed{mL}\ |\ 250\times5\ |\ 1250}{|\ 125\ \cancel{mg}\ |\ 125\ |\ 125} = 10\ mL$$

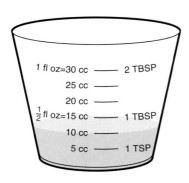

15. Sequential method:

$$\frac{200\ \cancel{mg}\ |\ \boxed{capsules}\ |\ 2}{|\ 100\ \cancel{mg}\ |\ 1} = 2\ capsules$$

16. Sequential method:

$$\frac{10\ \cancel{mg}\ |\ \boxed{tablet}\ |\ 10}{|\ 5\ \cancel{mg}\ |\ 5} = 2\ tablets$$

17. Sequential method:

$$\frac{3\ \cancel{mg}\ |\ \boxed{mL}\ |\ 3}{|\ 2\ \cancel{mg}\ |\ 2} = 1.5\ mL$$

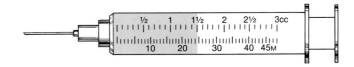

18. Sequential method:

$$\frac{400\ \cancel{mg}\ |\ 10.15\ \boxed{mL}\ |\ 400\times10.15\ |\ 4060}{|\ 325\ \cancel{mg}\ |\ 325\ |\ 325} = \begin{array}{c}12.49\ or\\12.5\ mL\end{array}$$

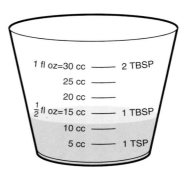

19. Random method:

$$\frac{\cancel{1000\ mg}\ |\ 2\ \boxed{mL}\ |\ 1\ \cancel{g}\ |\ 2\times1\ |\ 2}{|\ 1\ \cancel{g}\ |\ \cancel{1000\ mg}\ |\ 1\ |\ 1} = 2\ mL$$

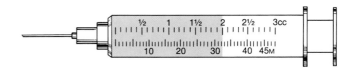

20. Sequential method:

$$\frac{10 \text{ mg}}{} \frac{5 \text{ mL}}{5 \text{ mg}} \frac{1 \text{ (tsp)}}{5 \text{ mL}} \frac{10 \times 1}{5} \frac{10}{5} = 2 \text{ tsp}$$

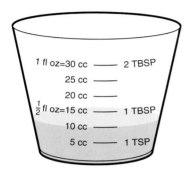

21. Random method:

$$\frac{0.25 \text{ mg}}{} \frac{\text{(mL)}}{250 \text{ mcg}} \frac{1000 \text{ mcg}}{1 \text{ mg}} \frac{0.25 \times 100}{25 \times 1} \frac{25}{25} = 1 \text{ mL}$$

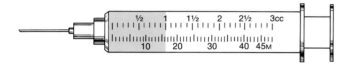

22. Sequential method:

$$\frac{500 \text{ mg}}{} \frac{\text{(mL)}}{300 \text{ mg}} \frac{5}{3} = 1.66 \text{ or } 1.7 \text{ mL}$$

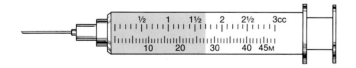

23. Sequential method:

$$\frac{2500 \text{ IU}}{} \frac{0.2 \text{ (mL)}}{2500 \text{ IU}} \frac{0.2}{} = 0.2 \text{ mL}$$

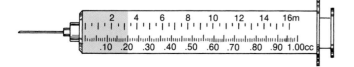

24. Sequential method:

$$\frac{200 \text{ mg}}{} \frac{5 \text{ (mL)}}{50 \text{ mg}} \frac{20 \times 5}{5} \frac{100}{5} = 20 \text{ mL}$$

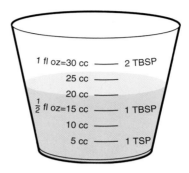

25. Sequential method:

$$\frac{300 \text{ mg}}{} \frac{\text{(capsule)}}{150 \text{ mg}} \frac{30}{15} = 2 \text{ capsules}$$

26. Sequential method:

$$\frac{500 \text{ mg}}{} \frac{\text{(tablets)}}{500 \text{ mg}} \frac{500}{500} = 1 \text{ tablet}$$

27. Sequential method:

$$\frac{0.25 \text{ mg}}{} \frac{\text{(tablets)}}{0.125 \text{ mg}} \frac{0.25}{0.125} = 2 \text{ tablets}$$

28. Sequential method:

$$\frac{25 \text{ mg}}{} \frac{\text{(tablets)}}{50 \text{ mg}} \frac{25}{50} = 0.5 \text{ tablet}$$

29. Sequential method:

$$\frac{5 \text{ mg}}{} \frac{\text{(tablets)}}{2.5 \text{ mg}} \frac{5}{2.5} = 2 \text{ tablets}$$

30. Sequential method:

$$\frac{0.5 \text{ mg}}{} \frac{\text{(tablets)}}{0.25 \text{ mg}} \frac{0.5}{0.25} = 2 \text{ tablets}$$

31. Sequential method:

$$\frac{150\ \cancel{mg}\ |\ \boxed{mL}\ |\ 15}{|\ 400\ \cancel{mg}\ |\ 40} = 0.375 \text{ or } 0.4 \text{ mL}$$

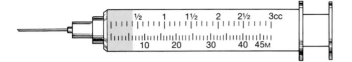

32. Sequential method:

$$\frac{600\ \cancel{mg}\ |\ \boxed{tablets}\ |\ 6}{|\ 300\ \cancel{mg}\ |\ 3} = 2 \text{ tablets}$$

Two-Factor Practice Problems

1. Random method:

$$\frac{25\ \cancel{mcg}\ |\ 2.5\ \boxed{mL}\ |\ 1\ \cancel{kg}\ |\ 1\ \cancel{mg}\ |\ 25\ \cancel{lb}}{\cancel{kg}\ |\ 0.125\ \cancel{mg}\ |\ 2.2\ \cancel{lb}\ |\ 1000\ \cancel{mcg}} = \text{mL}$$

$$\frac{25 \times 2.5 \times 1 \times 1 \times 25\ |\ 1562.5}{0.125 \times 2.2 \times 1000\ |\ 275} = 5.68 \text{ or } 5.7 \text{ mL}$$

2. Sequential method:

$$\frac{0.02\ \cancel{mg}\ |\ \boxed{mL}\ |\ 1\ \cancel{kg}\ |\ 35\ \cancel{lb}\ |\ 0.02 \times 1 \times 35\ |\ 0.7}{\cancel{kg}\ |\ 0.1\ \cancel{mg}\ |\ 2.2\ \cancel{lb}\ |\ |\ 0.1 \times 2.2\ |\ 0.22} = \frac{3.18 \text{ or}}{3.2 \text{ mL}}$$

3. Random method:

$$\frac{2\ \cancel{mg}\ |\ 500\ \boxed{mL}\ |\ 1\ \cancel{g}\ |\ 60\ \cancel{min}\ |\ 5 \times 6\ |\ 30}{\cancel{min}\ |\ 2\ \cancel{g}\ |\ 1000\ \cancel{mg}\ |\ 1\ \boxed{hr}\ |\ 1\ |\ 1} = \frac{30\ \text{mL}}{\text{hr}}$$

4. Sequential method:

$$\frac{1.5\ \cancel{g}\ |\ 10\ \boxed{mL}\ |\ 1.5 \times 10\ |\ 15}{|\ 1\ \cancel{g}\ |\ 1\ |\ 1} = 15 \text{ mL}$$

5. Sequential method:

$$\frac{1\ \cancel{mg}\ |\ \boxed{mL}\ |\ 1\ \cancel{kg}\ |\ 94\ \cancel{lb}\ |\ 1 \times 1 \times 94\ |\ 94}{\cancel{kg}\ |\ 40\ \cancel{mg}\ |\ 2.2\ \cancel{lb}\ |\ |\ 40 \times 2.2\ |\ 88} = \frac{1.068 \text{ or}}{1.1 \text{ mL}}$$

6. Sequential method:

$$\frac{15\ \cancel{mg}\ |\ 500\ \boxed{mL}\ |\ 15 \times 5\ |\ 75}{\boxed{hr}\ |\ 300\ \cancel{mg}\ |\ 3\ |\ 3} = \frac{25\ \text{mL}}{\text{hr}}$$

7. Sequential method:

$$\frac{25\ \cancel{mL}\ |\ 50\ \boxed{mg}\ |\ 5}{\boxed{hr}\ |\ 250\ \cancel{mL}\ |\ } = \frac{5\ \text{mg}}{\text{hr}}$$

8. Sequential method:

$$\frac{10\ \cancel{mEq}\ |\ 20\ \boxed{mL}\ |\ 10}{|\ 20\ \cancel{mEq}\ |\ } = 10 \text{ mL}$$

9. Sequential method:

$$\frac{3\ \cancel{mL}\ |\ 50\ \cancel{mg}\ |\ 1000\ \boxed{mcg}\ |\ 1\ \cancel{hr}\ |\ 3 \times 10\ |\ 30}{\cancel{hr}\ |\ 500\ \cancel{mL}\ |\ 1\ \cancel{mg}\ |\ 60\ \boxed{min}\ |\ 6\ |\ 6} = \frac{5\ \text{mcg}}{\text{min}}$$

10. Sequential method:

$$\frac{100\ \cancel{mL}\ |\ 10\ \boxed{mEq}\ |\ 1}{\boxed{hr}\ |\ 1000\ \cancel{mL}\ |\ } = \frac{1\ \text{mEq}}{\text{hr}}$$

11. Sequential method:

$$\frac{250\ \cancel{mL}\ |\ 20\ \boxed{gtt}\ |\ 1\ \cancel{hr}\ |\ 250 \times 2 \times 1\ |\ 500}{\cancel{hr}\ |\ \cancel{mL}\ |\ 60\ \boxed{min}\ |\ 6\ |\ 6} = \frac{83.3 \text{ or } 83 \text{ gtt}}{\text{min}}$$

12. Sequential method:

$$\frac{750\ \cancel{mL}\ |\ 10\ \boxed{gtt}\ |\ 1\ \cancel{hr}\ |\ 750 \times 1 \times 1\ |\ 750}{5\ \cancel{hr}\ |\ \cancel{mL}\ |\ 60\ \boxed{min}\ |\ 5 \times 6\ |\ 30} = \frac{25\ \text{gtt}}{\text{min}}$$

13. Sequential method:

$$\frac{500\ \cancel{mL}\ |\ 60\ \boxed{gtt}\ |\ 1\ \cancel{hr}\ |\ 500 \times 1\ |\ 500}{8\ \cancel{hr}\ |\ \cancel{mL}\ |\ 60\ \boxed{min}\ |\ 8\ |\ 8} = \frac{62.5 \text{ or } 63 \text{ gtt}}{\text{min}}$$

14. Sequential method:

$$\frac{750\ \cancel{mL}\ |\ 15\ \cancel{gtt}\ |\ \cancel{min}\ |\ 1\ \boxed{hr}\ |\ 750 \times 15 \times 1\ |\ 11250}{\cancel{mL}\ |\ 18\ \cancel{gtt}\ |\ 60\ \cancel{min}\ |\ 18 \times 60\ |\ 1080} = \frac{10.41 \text{ or}}{10 \text{ hr}}$$

15. Sequential method:

250 mL	15 gtt	min	1 hr	25 × 15 × 1	375	= 1.25 or
	mL	50 gtt	60 min	50 × 6	300	1 hr

16. Sequential method:

1000 mL	15 gtt	min	1 hr	100 × 15 × 1	1500	= 10 hr
	mL	25 gtt	60 min	25 × 6	150	

17. How many milliliters will you draw from the vial after reconstitution?
Sequential method:

$$\frac{1.25 \text{ g} \mid 10 \text{ mL} \mid 1.25 \times 10 \mid 12.5}{1 \text{ g} \mid 1 \mid 1} = 12.5 \text{ mL}$$

Calculate the milliliters per hour to set the IV pump.
Sequential method:

$$\frac{112.5 \text{ mL}}{\text{hr}} = 112.5 \text{ or } \frac{113 \text{ mL}}{\text{hr}}$$

Calculate the drops per minute with a drop factor of 10 gtt/mL.
Sequential method:

112.5 mL	10 gtt	1 hr	112.5 × 1 × 1	112.5	18.75 or 19 gtt
hr	mL	60 min	6	6	min

18. How many milliliters will you draw from the vial after reconstitution?
Sequential method:

$$\frac{275 \text{ mg} \mid 10 \text{ mL} \mid 275 \times 1 \mid 275}{500 \text{ mg} \mid 50 \mid 50} = 5.5 \text{ mL}$$

Calculate the milliliters per hour to set the IV pump.
Sequential method:

$$\frac{255.5 \text{ mL}}{\text{hr}} = 255.5 \text{ or } \frac{256 \text{ mL}}{\text{hr}}$$

Calculate the drops per minute with a drop factor of 10 gtt/mL.
Sequential method:

255.5 mL	10 gtt	1 hr	255.5 × 1 × 1	255.5	42.5 or 43 gtt
hr	mL	60 min	6	6	min

19. How many milliliters will you draw from the vial after reconstitution?
Random method:

450 mg	10 mL	1 g	45 × 1	45	= 4.5 mL
	1 g	1000 mg	10	10	

Calculate the milliliters per hour to set the IV pump.
Sequential method:

104.5 mL	60 min	104.5 × 6	627	209 mL
30 min	1 hr	3 × 1	3	hr

Calculate the drops per minute with a drop factor of 10 gtt/mL.
Sequential method:

104.5 mL	10 gtt	104.5 × 1	104.5	34.8 or 35 gtt
30 min	mL	3	3	min

20. How many milliliters will you draw from the vial?
Sequential method:

$$\frac{23 \text{ mg} \mid \text{mL} \mid 23}{40 \text{ mg} \mid 40} = 0.57 \text{ or } 0.6 \text{ mL}$$

Calculate the milliliters per hour to set the IV pump.
Sequential method:

$$\frac{100.6 \text{ mL}}{\text{hr}} = 100.6 \text{ or } \frac{101 \text{ mL}}{\text{hr}}$$

Calculate the drops per minute with a drop factor of 15 gtt/mL.

100.6 mL	15 gtt	1 hr	100.6 × 15 × 1	1509	25.15 or 25 gtt
hr	mL	60 min	60	60	min

21. Sequential method:

0.56 mg	18 kg	5 mL	0.56 × 18 × 5	50.4
kg		10 mg	10	10

= 5.04 or 5 mL

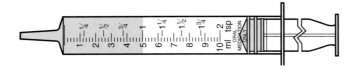

22. Random method:

30 g	day	packet	30	30
day	4 doses	5 g	4 × 5	20

= $\dfrac{1.5 \text{ packet}}{\text{dose}}$

23. Random method:

10 mcg	2 mL	50 kg	1 mg	1 × 2 × 5 × 1	10
kg	2 mg		1000 mcg	2 × 10	20

= 0.5 mL

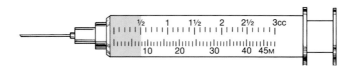

24. Sequential method:

1600 mg	tablets	day	16	16
day	800 mg	2 doses	8 × 2	16

= $\dfrac{1 \text{ tablet}}{\text{dose}}$

25. Random method:

1 g	mL	1000 mg	day	10	10
day	100 mg	1 g	3 doses	1 × 3	

= $\dfrac{3.33 \text{ or } 3 \text{ mL}}{\text{dose}}$

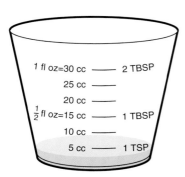

26. Sequential method:

4 mg	mL	20 kg	4 × 2	8
kg	10 mg		1	1

= 8 mL

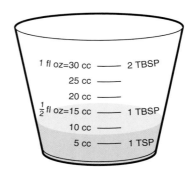

27. Sequential method:

0.15 mg	mL	1 kg	160 lb	0.15 × 1 × 160	24
kg	2 mg	2.2 lb		2 × 2.2	4.4

= 5.45 or 5.5 mL

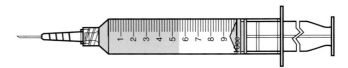

28. Sequential method:

2 mg	tablets	40 kg	2 × 4	8
kg	150 mg		15	15

= 0.533 or 0.5 tablet

29. Sequential method:

20 mg	tablet	1 kg	20 lb	2 × 1 × 2	4
kg	400 mg	2.2 lb		4 × 2.2	8.8

= 0.45 or 0.5 tablet

30. Sequential method:

450 mg	tablet	day	45	45
day	150 mg	3 doses	15 × 3	45

= $\dfrac{1 \text{ tablet}}{\text{dose}}$

31. Random method:

$$\frac{2.4\ \cancel{g}}{\cancel{day}} \left| \frac{\cancel{(tablet)}}{300\ \cancel{mg}} \right| \frac{\cancel{day}}{4\ \cancel{(doses)}} \left| \frac{1000\ \cancel{mg}}{1\ \cancel{g}} \right| \frac{2.4 \times 10}{3 \times 4 \times 1} \left| \frac{24}{12} \right| = \frac{2\ tablets}{dose}$$

32. Sequential method:

$$\frac{500\ \cancel{mg}}{\cancel{day}} \left| \frac{8\ \cancel{(mL)}}{750\ \cancel{mg}} \right| \frac{\cancel{day}}{2\ \cancel{(doses)}} \left| \frac{50 \times 8}{75 \times 2} \right| \frac{400}{150} = \frac{2.666\ or}{2.7\ mL} \over dose$$

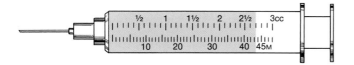

33. Random method:

$$\frac{1000\ \cancel{mg}}{\cancel{day}} \left| \frac{20\ \cancel{(mL)}}{2\ \cancel{g}} \right| \frac{1\ \cancel{g}}{1000\ \cancel{mg}} \left| \frac{\cancel{day}}{2\ \cancel{(doses)}} \right| \frac{20 \times 1}{2 \times 2} \left| \frac{20}{4} \right| = \frac{5\ mL}{dose}$$

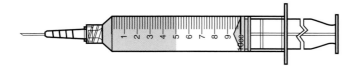

Three-Factor Practice Problems

1. How many milliliters per day will you give?
Sequential method:

$$\frac{40\ \cancel{mg}}{\cancel{kg}/\cancel{(day)}} \left| \frac{5\ \cancel{(mL)}}{300\ \cancel{mg}} \right| 60\ \cancel{kg} \left| \frac{4 \times 5 \times 6}{3} \right| \frac{120}{3} = \frac{40\ mL}{day}$$

How many milliliters per dose will you give?
Sequential method:

$$\frac{40\ \cancel{mg}}{\cancel{kg}/\cancel{day}} \left| \frac{5\ \cancel{(mL)}}{300\ \cancel{mg}} \right| 60\ \cancel{kg} \left| \frac{\cancel{day}}{4\ \cancel{(doses)}} \right| \frac{4 \times 5 \times 6}{3 \times 4} \left| \frac{120}{12} \right| = \frac{10\ mL}{dose}$$

2. Sequential method:

$$\frac{4\ \cancel{mg}}{\cancel{kg}/\cancel{(day)}} \left| \frac{\cancel{(mL)}}{10\ \cancel{mg}} \right| \frac{1\ \cancel{kg}}{2.2\ \cancel{lb}} \left| 60\ \cancel{lb} \right| \frac{4 \times 1 \times 6}{1 \times 2.2} \left| \frac{24}{2.2} \right| = \frac{10.9\ or\ 11\ mL}{day}$$

3. How many milliliters per day will you give?
Sequential method:

$$\frac{30\ \cancel{mg}}{\cancel{kg}/\cancel{(day)}} \left| \frac{2\ \cancel{(mL)}}{300\ \cancel{mg}} \right| 50\ \cancel{kg} \left| \frac{2 \times 5}{} \right| \frac{10}{} = \frac{10\ mL}{day}$$

How many milliliters per dose will you give?
Sequential method:

$$\frac{30\ \cancel{mg}}{\cancel{kg}/\cancel{day}} \left| \frac{2\ \cancel{(mL)}}{300\ \cancel{mg}} \right| 50\ \cancel{kg} \left| \frac{\cancel{day}}{3\ \cancel{(doses)}} \right| \frac{2 \times 5}{3} \left| \frac{10}{3} \right| = \frac{3.33\ or\ 3.3\ mL}{dose}$$

4. Sequential method:

$$\frac{0.575\ \cancel{mL}}{\cancel{dose}} \left| \frac{40\ \cancel{(mg)}}{mL} \right| \frac{2.2\ \cancel{lb}}{1\ \cancel{(kg)}} \left| \frac{}{45\ \cancel{lb}} \right| \frac{3\ \cancel{doses}}{\cancel{(day)}} = \frac{mg}{kg/day}$$

$$\frac{0.575 \times 40 \times 2.2 \times 3}{1 \times 45} \left| \frac{151.8}{45} \right| = \frac{3.37\ or\ 3.4}{} \frac{mg}{kg/day}$$

5. Sequential method:

$$\frac{0.125\ \cancel{mL}}{\cancel{dose}} \left| \frac{50\ \cancel{(mg)}}{mL} \right| \frac{2.2\ \cancel{lb}}{1\ \cancel{(kg)}} \left| \frac{}{20\ \cancel{lb}} \right| \frac{3\ \cancel{doses}}{\cancel{(day)}} = \frac{mg}{kg/day}$$

$$\frac{0.125 \times 5 \times 2.2 \times 3}{1 \times 2} \left| \frac{4.125}{2} \right| = \frac{2.06\ or\ 2.1}{} \frac{mg}{kg/day}$$

6. How many milliliters will you draw from the vial?
Sequential method:

$$\frac{400\ \cancel{mg}}{} \left| \frac{10\ \cancel{(mL)}}{400\ \cancel{mg}} \right| \frac{10}{} = 10\ mL$$

Calculate the milliliters per hour to set the IV pump.
Random method:

$$\frac{5\ \cancel{mcg}}{\cancel{kg}/\cancel{min}} \left| \frac{260\ \cancel{(mL)}}{400\ \cancel{mg}} \right| \frac{1\ \cancel{mg}}{1000\ \cancel{mcg}} \left| \frac{\cancel{kg}}{2.2\ \cancel{lb}} \right| 110\ \cancel{lb} \left| \frac{60\ \cancel{min}}{\cancel{(hr)}} \right| = \frac{mL}{hr}$$

$$\frac{5 \times 26 \times 1 \times 11 \times 6}{4 \times 100 \times 2.2} \left| \frac{8580}{880} \right| = \frac{9.75\ or\ 9.8\ mL}{hr}$$

7. Random method:

0.8 mcg	500 mL	1 mg	1 kg	60 min	143 lb	= mL
kg/min	50 mg	1000 mcg	2.2 lb	1 hr		hr

$$\frac{0.8 \times 5 \times 1 \times 6 \times 143}{5 \times 10 \times 2.2} \left| \frac{3432}{110} \right. = \frac{31.2 \text{ mL}}{\text{hr}}$$

8. Sequential method:

68 mL	50 mg	1 hr	2.2 lb	1000 mcg		= mcg
hr	250 mL	60 min	1 kg	1 mg	250 lb	kg/min

$$\frac{68 \times 5 \times 1 \times 2.2 \times 10}{25 \times 6 \times 1 \times 1 \times 25} \left| \frac{7480}{3750} \right. = 1.99 \text{ or } 2 \frac{\text{mcg}}{\text{kg/min}}$$

9. Random method:

30 mg	1 kg	157 lb	1 g	3 × 1 × 157 × 1	471	2.14 or 2.1 g
kg/day	2.2 lb		1000 mg	2.2 × 100	220 =	day

10. Random method:

0.01 mL	1 kg	180 lb	60 min	0.01 × 1× 180 × 60
kg/min	2.2 lb		1 hr	2.2 × 1

$$\frac{108}{2.2} = \frac{49.09 \text{ or } 49.1 \text{ mL}}{\text{hr}}$$

11. Random method:

28 mL	400 mg		1 hr	1000 mcg	= mcg
hr	250 mL	15 kg	60 min	1 mg	kg/min

$$\frac{28 \times 4 \times 1 \times 1000}{25 \times 15 \times 6 \times 1} \left| \frac{112{,}000}{2250} \right. = 49.77 \text{ or } 49.8 \frac{\text{mcg}}{\text{kg/min}}$$

12. Random method:

3 mcg	100 mL	1 kg	60 min	160 lb	1 mg	= mL
kg/min	100 mg	2.2 lb	1 hr		1000 mcg	hr

$$\frac{3 \times 1 \times 6 \times 16 \times 1}{2.2 \times 1 \times 10} \left| \frac{288}{22} \right. = 13.09 \text{ or } 13.1 \frac{\text{mL}}{\text{hr}}$$

13. Random method:

2 mcg	250 mL	1 kg	250 lb	1 mg	60 min
kg/min	50 mg	2.2 lb		1000 mcg	1 hr

$$\frac{2 \times 25 \times 1 \times 25 \times 6}{5 \times 2.2 \times 10} \left| \frac{7500}{110} \right. = 68.1 \text{ or } \frac{68 \text{ mL}}{\text{hr}}$$

14. Random method:

1 mcg	250 mL	1 kg	60 min	160 lb	1 mg	= mL
kg/min	50 mg	2.2 lb	1 hr		1000 mcg	hr

$$\frac{1 \times 25 \times 6 \times 16}{50 \times 2.2} \left| \frac{2400}{110} \right. = 21.81 \text{ or } 21.8 \frac{\text{mL}}{\text{hr}}$$

15. Random method:

2.5 mcg	500 mL	65 kg	60 min	1 mg	= mL
kg/min	400 mg		1 hr	1000 mcg	hr

$$\frac{2.5 \times 5 \times 65 \times 6 \times 1}{4 \times 1 \times 100} \left| \frac{4875}{400} \right. = 12.18 \text{ or } 12.2 \frac{\text{mL}}{\text{hr}}$$

16. Random method:

15 mL	2 mg	1 hr		1000 mcg	= mcg
hr	500 mL	60 min	20 kg	1 mg	kg/min

$$\frac{15 \times 2 \times 1 \times 1}{5 \times 6 \times 20 \times 1} \left| \frac{30}{600} \right. = 0.05 \frac{\text{mcg}}{\text{kg/min}}$$

17. Random method:

$$\frac{5 \ \cancel{mcg}}{\cancel{kg}/\cancel{min}} \ \Big| \ \frac{500 \ \textcircled{mL}}{400 \ mg} \ \Big| \ \frac{70 \ \cancel{kg}}{} \ \Big| \ \frac{1 \ \cancel{mg}}{1000 \ \cancel{mcg}} = \frac{mL}{min}$$

$$\frac{5 \times 5 \times 7 \times 1}{4 \times 100} \ \Big| \ \frac{175}{400} = \frac{0.4375 \ \text{or} \ 0.44 \ mL}{min}$$

18. How many milligrams per day is the child receiving?
    Sequential method:

$$\frac{40 \ \textcircled{mg}}{\cancel{kg}/\textcircled{day}} \ \Big| \ \frac{1 \ \cancel{kg}}{2.2 \ \cancel{lb}} \ \Big| \ \frac{20 \ \cancel{lb}}{} \ \Big| \ \frac{40 \times 1 \times 20}{2.2} \ \Big| \ \frac{800}{2.2} = \frac{363.63 \ \text{or} \ 363.6 \ mg}{day}$$

How many milligrams per dose is the child receiving?
Sequential method:

$$\frac{363.6 \ \textcircled{mg}}{\cancel{day}} \ \Big| \ \frac{\cancel{day}}{3 \ \textcircled{doses}} \ \Big| \ \frac{363.6}{3} = \frac{121.2 \ mg}{dose}$$

How many milliliters will you draw from the vial after reconstitution?
Sequential method:

$$\frac{121.2 \ \cancel{mg}}{} \ \Big| \ \frac{10 \ \textcircled{mL}}{500 \ \cancel{mg}} \ \Big| \ \frac{121.2 \times 10}{500} \ \Big| \ \frac{1212}{500} = 2.424 \ \text{or} \ 2.4 \ mL$$

Calculate the milliliters per hour to set the IV pump.
Sequential method:

$$\frac{102.4 \ \textcircled{mL}}{60 \ \cancel{min}} \ \Big| \ \frac{60 \ \cancel{min}}{1 \ \textcircled{hr}} \ \Big| \ \frac{102.4}{1} = \frac{102.4 \ mL}{hr}$$

19. How many milligrams per dose is the child receiving?
    Random method:

$$\frac{2 \ \textcircled{mg}}{\cancel{kg}/\textcircled{dose}} \ \Big| \ \frac{40 \ \cancel{kg}}{} \ \Big| \ \frac{2 \times 40}{} \ \Big| \ \frac{80}{} = \frac{80 \ mg}{dose}$$

How many milliliters will you draw from the vial?
Sequential method:

$$\frac{80 \ \cancel{mg}}{} \ \Big| \ \frac{\textcircled{mL}}{40 \ \cancel{mg}} \ \Big| \ \frac{8}{4} = 2 \ mL$$

Calculate the milliliters per hour to set the IV pump.
Sequential method:

$$\frac{52 \ \textcircled{mL}}{30 \ \cancel{min}} \ \Big| \ \frac{60 \ \cancel{min}}{1 \ \textcircled{hr}} \ \Big| \ \frac{52 \times 6}{3 \times 1} \ \Big| \ \frac{312}{3} = \frac{104 \ mL}{hr}$$

20. How many milligrams per day is the child receiving?
    Sequential method:

$$\frac{25 \ \textcircled{mg}}{\cancel{kg}/\textcircled{day}} \ \Big| \ \frac{25 \ \cancel{kg}}{} \ \Big| \ \frac{25 \times 25}{} \ \Big| \ \frac{625}{} = \frac{625 \ mg}{day}$$

How many milligrams per dose is the child receiving?
Sequential method:

$$\frac{625 \ \textcircled{mg}}{\cancel{day}} \ \Big| \ \frac{\cancel{day}}{3 \ \textcircled{doses}} \ \Big| \ \frac{625}{3} = \frac{208.33 \ \text{or} \ 208.3 \ mg}{dose}$$

How many milliliters will you draw from the vial after reconstitution?
Sequential method:

$$\frac{208.3 \ \cancel{mg}}{} \ \Big| \ \frac{10 \ \textcircled{mL}}{500 \ \cancel{mg}} \ \Big| \ \frac{208.3 \times 1}{50} \ \Big| \ \frac{208.3}{50} = \frac{4.166 \ \text{or} \ 4.2 \ mL}{day}$$

Calculate the milliliters per hour to set the IV pump.
Sequential method:

$$\frac{54.2 \ \textcircled{mL}}{30 \ min} \ \Big| \ \frac{60 \ min}{1 \ \textcircled{hr}} \ \Big| \ \frac{54.2 \times 6}{3 \times 1} \ \Big| \ \frac{325.2}{3} = \frac{108.4 \ mL}{hr}$$

Comprehensive Practice Problems

1. Sequential method:

$$\frac{0.125 \text{ mg} \mid \text{(tablet)} \mid 0.125}{0.25 \text{ mg} \mid 0.25} = 0.5 \text{ tablet}$$

Answer: 0.5 tablet

2. Random method:

$$\frac{0.5 \text{ g} \mid \text{(tablet)} \mid 1000 \text{ mg} \mid 0.5 \times 10 \mid 5}{500 \text{ mg} \mid 1 \text{ g} \mid 5 \times 1 \mid 5} = 1 \text{ tablet}$$

Answer: 1 tablet

3. Random method:

$$\frac{\frac{1}{150} \text{ gr} \mid \text{(mL)} \mid 60 \text{ mg} \mid \frac{1}{150} \times \frac{60}{1} \mid \frac{60}{150} \mid 0.4}{0.4 \text{ mg} \mid 1 \text{ gr} \mid 0.4 \times 1 \mid 0.4 \mid 0.4} = 1 \text{ mL}$$

Answer: 1 mL

4. Sequential method:

$$\frac{500{,}000 \text{ units} \mid \text{mL} \mid 1 \text{ (tsp)} \mid 5 \times 1 \mid 5}{100{,}000 \text{ units} \mid 5 \text{ mL} \mid 1 \times 5 \mid 5} = 1 \text{ tsp}$$

Answer: 1 tsp

5. Sequential method:

$$\frac{50 \text{ mg} \mid \text{(mL)} \mid 5}{100 \text{ mg} \mid 10} = 0.5 \text{ mL}$$

Answer: 0.5 mL

6. Sequential method:

$$\frac{2 \text{ mg} \mid 10 \text{ (mL)} \mid 75 \text{ kg} \mid 2 \times 1 \times 75 \mid 150}{\text{kg} \mid 500 \text{ mg} \mid \mid 50 \mid 50} = 3 \text{ mL}$$

Answer: 3 mL

7. Sequential method:

$$\frac{2 \text{ mg} \mid 5 \text{ (mL)} \mid 1 \text{ kg} \mid 100 \text{ lb} \mid 2 \times 5 \times 1 \times 1 \mid 10}{\text{kg} \mid 500 \text{ mg} \mid 2.2 \text{ lb} \mid \mid 5 \times 2.2 \mid 11} = 0.9 \text{ mL}$$

Answer: 0.9 mL

8. Sequential method:

$$\frac{1000 \text{ mL} \mid 15 \text{ (gtt)} \mid 1 \text{ hr} \mid 100 \times 15 \times 1 \mid 1500}{12 \text{ hr} \mid \text{mL} \mid 60 \text{ (min)} \mid 12 \times 6 \mid 72} = 20.8 \text{ or } 21 \frac{\text{gtt}}{\text{min}}$$

Answer: 21 gtt/min

9. Sequential method:

$$\frac{500 \text{ mL} \mid 15 \text{ gtt} \mid \text{min} \mid 1 \text{ (hr)} \mid 50 \times 15 \times 1 \mid 750}{\text{mL} \mid 21 \text{ gtt} \mid 60 \text{ min} \mid 21 \times 6 \mid 126} = 5.9 \text{ hr}$$

Answer: 5.9 hours (Do not round up due to pump)

10. Sequential method:

$$\frac{1500 \text{ units} \mid 250 \text{ (mL)} \mid 15 \times 25 \mid 375}{\text{(hr)} \mid 25{,}000 \text{ units} \mid 25 \mid 25} = 15 \frac{\text{mL}}{\text{hr}}$$

Answer: 15 mL/hr

11. Sequential method:

$$\frac{1000 \text{ mL} \mid 15 \text{ gtt} \mid \text{min} \mid 1 \text{ (hr)} \mid 10 \times 15 \times 1 \mid 150}{\text{mL} \mid 50 \text{ gtt} \mid 60 \text{ min} \mid 5 \times 6 \mid 30} = 5 \text{ hr}$$

Answer: 5 hours

12. Sequential method:

$$\frac{8 \text{ units} \mid 250 \text{ (mL)} \mid 8 \times 25 \mid 200}{\text{(hr)} \mid 100 \text{ units} \mid 10 \mid 10} = 20 \frac{\text{mL}}{\text{hr}}$$

Answer: 20 mL/hr

13. Sequential method:

$$\frac{500\ \text{mL}}{8\ \text{hr}}\left|\frac{10\ \text{gtt}}{\text{mL}}\right|\frac{1\ \text{hr}}{60\ \text{min}}\left|\frac{50\times10\times1}{8\times6}\right|\frac{500}{48}=\frac{10.4\ \text{or}\ 10\ \text{gtt}}{\text{min}}$$

Answer: 10 gtt/min

14. Random method:

$$\frac{2\ \text{mEq}}{100\ \text{mL}}\left|\frac{10\ \text{mL}}{20\ \text{mEq}}\right|\frac{500\ \text{mL}}{}\left|\frac{2\times1\times5}{1\times2}\right|\frac{10}{2}=5\ \text{mL}$$

Answer: 5 mL

15. Random method:

$$\frac{44\ \text{mg}}{\text{hr}}\left|\frac{250\ \text{mL}}{1\ \text{g}}\right|\frac{1\ \text{g}}{1000\ \text{mg}}\left|\frac{44\times25\times1}{1\times100}\right|\frac{1100}{100}=\frac{11\ \text{mL}}{\text{hr}}$$

Answer: 11 mL/hr

16. Sequential method:

$$\frac{140\ \text{mL}}{\text{hr}}\left|\frac{30\ \text{mg}}{1000\ \text{mL}}\right|\frac{14\times3}{10}\left|\frac{42}{10}\right.=\frac{4.2\ \text{mg}}{\text{hr}}$$

Answer: 4.2 mg/hr

17. How many milliliters will you draw from the vial after reconstitution?
Sequential method:

$$\frac{750\ \text{mg}}{}\left|\frac{\text{mL}}{500\ \text{mg}}\right|\frac{75}{50}=1.5\ \text{mL}$$

Calculate the milliliters per hour to set the IV pump.
Sequential method:

$$\frac{101.5\ \text{mL}}{30\ \text{min}}\left|\frac{60\ \text{min}}{1\ \text{hr}}\right|\frac{101.5\times6}{3\times1}\left|\frac{609}{3}\right.=\frac{203\ \text{mL}}{\text{hr}}$$

Calculate the drops per minute with a drop factor of 10 gtt/mL.
Sequential method:

$$\frac{203\ \text{mL}}{\text{hr}}\left|\frac{10\ \text{gtt}}{\text{mL}}\right|\frac{1\ \text{hr}}{60\ \text{min}}\left|\frac{203\times1\times1}{6}\right|\frac{203}{6}=\frac{33.83\ \text{or}\ 34\ \text{gtt}}{\text{min}}$$

18. How many milliliters will you draw from the vial after reconstitution?
Sequential method:

$$\frac{1.5\ \text{g}}{3\ \text{g}}\left|\frac{5\ \text{mL}}{}\right|\frac{1.5\times5}{3}\left|\frac{7.5}{3}\right.=2.5\ \text{mL}$$

Calculate the milliliters per hour to set the IV pump.
Sequential method:

$$\frac{52.5\ \text{mL}}{20\ \text{min}}\left|\frac{60\ \text{min}}{1\ \text{hr}}\right|\frac{52.5\times6}{2\times1}\left|\frac{315}{2}\right.=\frac{157.5\ \text{or}\ 158\ \text{mL}}{\text{hr}}$$

Calculate the drops per minute with a drop factor of 20 gtt/mL.
Sequential method:

$$\frac{158\ \text{mL}}{\text{hr}}\left|\frac{20\ \text{gtt}}{\text{mL}}\right|\frac{1\ \text{hr}}{60\ \text{min}}\left|\frac{158\times2\times1}{6}\right|\frac{316}{6}=\frac{52.66\ \text{or}\ 53\ \text{gtt}}{\text{min}}$$

19. Random method:

$$\frac{4\ \text{mcg}}{\text{kg/min}}\left|\frac{250\ \text{mL}}{400\ \text{mg}}\right|\frac{1\ \text{mg}}{1000\ \text{mcg}}\left|\frac{60\ \text{min}}{1\ \text{hr}}\right|\frac{1\ \text{kg}}{2.2\ \text{lb}}\left|\frac{120\ \text{lb}}{}\right.=\frac{\text{mL}}{\text{hr}}$$

$$\frac{4\times25\times1\times6\times1\times12}{40\times10\times1\times2.2}\left|\frac{7200}{880}\right.=\frac{8.1\ \text{or}\ 8\ \text{mL}}{\text{hr}}$$

Answer: 8 mL/hr

20. Random method:

$$\frac{0.8\ \text{mcg}}{\text{kg/min}}\left|\frac{500\ \text{mL}}{50\ \text{mg}}\right|\frac{1\ \text{mg}}{1000\ \text{mcg}}\left|\frac{1\ \text{kg}}{2.2\ \text{lb}}\right|\frac{143\ \text{lb}}{}\left|\frac{60\ \text{min}}{1\ \text{hr}}\right.=\frac{\text{mL}}{\text{hr}}$$

$$\frac{0.8\times5\times1\times1\times143\times6}{5\times10\times2.2\times1}\left|\frac{3432}{110}\right.=\frac{31.2\ \text{or}\ 31\ \text{mL}}{\text{hr}}$$

Answer: 31 mL/hr

3

Case Studies

This section contains case studies simulating typical orders that might be written for patients with selected disorders. In each case, the orders include multiple situations that require the nurse to perform clinical calculations before being able to implement the order. After reading the short scenario, read through the list of orders.

Place a check mark in the box next to the physician's order that probably requires further calculations before implementing.

■ CASE STUDY 1   Congestive Heart Failure

A patient is admitted to the hospital with a diagnosis of dyspnea, peripheral edema with a 10-lb weight gain, and a history of congestive heart failure. The orders from the physician include:

- ❏ Bed rest in Fowler's position
- ❏ O_2 at 4 L/min per nasal cannula
- ❏ Chest x-ray, complete blood count, electrolyte panel, BUN, serum creatinine levels, and a digoxin level
- ❏ IV of D5W/$\frac{1}{2}$NS at 50 cc/hr
- ❏ Daily AM weight
- ❏ Antiembolism stockings
- ❏ Furosemide 40 mg IV qd
- ❏ Digoxin 0.125 mg PO qd
- ❏ KCl 20 mEq PO tid
- ❏ Low-Na diet
- ❏ Restrict PO fluids to 1500 cc/day
- ❏ Vitals q4h
- ❏ Accurate I/O

Identify the orders that require calculations.

Set up and solve each problem using dimensional analysis.

1. Calculate gtt/min using microtubing (60 gtt/mL).

2. Calculate the weight gain in kilograms.

3. Calculate how many mL of Lasix the patient will receive IV from a multi-dose vial labeled 10 mg/mL.

4. Calculate how many tablets of digoxin the patient will receive from a unit dose of 0.25 mg/tablet.

5. Calculate how many tablets of K-Dur the patient will receive from a unit dose of 10 mEq/tablet.

■ CASE STUDY 2   COPD/Emphysema

A patient is admitted to the hospital with dyspnea and COPD exacerbation. The orders from the physician include:

- ❏ Stat ABGs, chest x-ray, complete blood count, and electrolytes
- ❏ IV D5W/$\frac{1}{2}$ NS 1000 cc/8 hr
- ❏ Aminophylline IV loading dose of 5.6 mg/kg over 30 minutes followed by 0.5 mg/kg/hr continuous IV
- ❏ O_2 at 2 L/min per nasal cannula
- ❏ Albuterol respiratory treatments q4h
- ❏ Chest physiotherapy q4h
- ❏ Erythromycin 800 mg IV q6h
- ❏ Bed rest
- ❏ Accurate I/O
- ❏ High-calorie, protein-rich diet in six small meals daily
- ❏ Encourage PO fluids to 3 L/day

Identify the orders that require calculations.

Set up and solve each problem using dimensional analysis.

1. Calculate cc/hr to set the IV pump.

2. Calculate cc/hr to set the IV pump for the loading dose of aminophylline for a patient weighing 140 lb. Aminophylline supply: 100 mg/100 mL D5W.

3. Calculate cc/hr to set the IV pump for the continuous dose of amino-phylline for a patient weighing 140 lb. Aminophylline supply: 1 g/250 mL D5W.

4. Calculate cc/hr to set the IV pump to infuse erythromycin 800 mg. Eryth-romycin supply: 1-g vial to be reconstituted with 20 mL sterile water and further diluted in 250 cc NS to infuse over 1 hr.

5. Calculate the PO fluids in mL/shift.

■ CASE STUDY 3   Small Cell Lung Cancer

A patient with small cell lung cancer is admitted to the hospital with fever and dehydration. The orders from the physician include:

- ❑ O$_2$ at 2 L/min per nasal cannula
- ❑ Chest x-ray; complete blood count; electrolytes; blood, urine, and sputum cultures; BUN and serum creatinine levels; type and cross for 2 units of PRBCs
- ❑ IV D5W/$\frac{1}{2}$ NS 1000 cc with 10 mEq KCl at 125 cc/hr
- ❑ 2 units of PRBCs if Hg is below 8
- ❑ 6 pack of platelets if <20,000
- ❑ Neupogen 5 mcg/kg SQ daily
- ❑ Gentamicin 80 mg IV q8h
- ❑ Decadron 8 mg IV daily
- ❑ Fortaz 1 g IV q8h
- ❑ Accurate I/O
- ❑ Encourage PO fluids
- ❑ Vitals q4h (call for temperature >102°F)

Identify the orders that require calculations.

Set up and solve each problem using dimensional analysis.

1. Calculate gtt/min using macrotubing (20 gtt/mL).

2. Calculate how many mcg of Neupogen will be given SQ to a patient weighing 160 lb.

3. Calculate cc/hr to set the IV pump to infuse gentamicin. The vial is labeled 40 mg/mL and is to be further diluted in 100 cc D5W to infuse over 1 hr.

4. Calculate how many mL of Decadron the patient will receive from a vial labeled dexamethasone 4 mg/mL.

5. Calculate mL/hr to set the IV pump to infuse Fortaz 1 g over 30 minutes. Supply: Fortaz 1 g/50 mL.

■ **CASE STUDY 4**   **Acquired Immunodeficiency Syndrome (AIDS)**

A patient who is HIV+ and a Jehovah's Witness is admitted to the hospital with anemia, fever of unknown origin, and wasting syndrome with dehydration. The orders from the physician include:

- ❏ O$_2$ at 4 L/min per nasal cannula
- ❏ IV D5W/$\frac{1}{2}$ NS at 150 cc/hr
- ❏ CD4 and CD8 T-cell subset counts; erythrocyte sedimentation rate; complete blood count; urine, sputum, and stool cultures; chest x-ray
- ❏ Acyclovir 350 mg IV q8h
- ❏ Neupogen 300 mcg SQ daily
- ❏ Epogen 100 units/kg SQ three times a week
- ❏ Megace 40 mg PO tid
- ❏ Zidovudine 100 mg PO q4h
- ❏ Vancomycin 800 mg IV q6h
- ❏ Respiratory treatments with pentamidine
- ❏ High-calorie, protein-rich diet in six small meals daily
- ❏ Encourage PO fluids to 3 L/day
- ❏ Accurate I/O
- ❏ Daily AM weight

Identify the orders that require calculations.

Set up and solve each problem using dimensional analysis.

1. Calculate gtt/min using macrotubing (20 gtt/mL).

2. Calculate cc/hr to set the IV pump to infuse acyclovir 350 mg. Supply: 500-mg vial to be reconstituted with 10 mL sterile water and further diluted in 100 mL D5W to infuse over 1 hr.

3. Calculate how many mL of Neupogen will be given SQ. The vial is labeled 300 mcg/mL.

4. Calculate how many mL of Epogen will be given SQ to the patient weighing 100 lb. The vial is labeled 4000 units/mL.

5. Calculate how many cc/hr to set the IV pump to infuse vancomycin 800 mg. Supply: 1-g vials to be reconstituted with 10 mL NS and further diluted in 100 mL D5W to infuse over 60 min.

■ CASE STUDY 5   Sickle Cell Anemia

A patient is admitted to the hospital in sickle cell crisis. The orders from the physician include:

❏ Bed rest with joint support
❏ O_2 at 2 L/min per nasal cannula
❏ Complete blood count, erythrocyte sedimentation rate, serum iron levels, and chest x-ray
❏ IV D5W/$\frac{1}{2}$ NS at 150 cc/hr
❏ Zofran 8 mg IV q8h
❏ Morphine sulfate 5 mg IV prn
❏ Hydrea 10 mg/kg/day PO
❏ Folic acid 0.5 mg daily PO
❏ Encourage 3000 cc/daily PO

Identify the orders that require calculations.

Set up and solve each problem using dimensional analysis.

1. Calculate gtt/min using macrotubing (10 gtt/mL).

2. Calculate cc/hr to set the IV pump to infuse Zofran 8 mg. Supply: Zofran 8 mg in 50 cc D5W to infuse over 15 min.

3. Calculate how many mL of morphine sulfate will be given IV. The syringe is labeled 10 mg/mL.

4. Calculate how many mg/day of Hydrea will be given PO to the patient weighing 125 lb.

5. Calculate how many tablets of folic acid will be given PO. Supply: 1 mg/tablet.

■ CASE STUDY 6   Deep Vein Thrombosis

A patient is admitted to the hospital with right leg erythema and edema to R/O DVT. The orders from the physician include:

❏ Bed rest with right leg elevated
❏ Warm, moist heat to right leg with Aqua-K pad
❏ Doppler ultrasonography
❏ Partial thromboplastin time (PTT) and prothrombin time (PT)
❏ IV D5W/$\frac{1}{2}$ NS with 20 mEq KCl at 50 cc/hr

❏ Heparin 5000 units IV push followed by continuous IV infusion of 1000 units/hr
❏ Lasix 20 mg IV bid
❏ Morphine 5 mg IV q4h

Identify the orders that require calculations.

Set up and solve each problem using dimensional analysis.

1. Calculate gtt/min using microtubing (60 gtt/mL).

2. Calculate how many mL of heparin the patient will receive IV from a multidose vial labeled 10,000 units/mL.

3. Calculate mL/hr to set the IV pump for the continuous dose of heparin. Heparin supply: 25,000 units/250 mL D5W.

4. Calculate how many mL of Lasix the patient will receive IV from a multidose vial labeled 10 mg/mL.

5. Calculate how many mL of morphine the patient will receive from a syringe labeled 10 mg/mL.

■ CASE STUDY 7   Bone Marrow Transplant

A patient is admitted to the hospital with a rash after an allogeneic bone marrow transplant. The orders from the physician include:

❏ IV D5W/$\frac{1}{2}$ NS with 20 mEq KCl/L at 80 cc/hr
❏ Complete blood count; electrolytes; sputum, urine, and stool cultures; blood cultures ×3; liver panel; BUN; and creatinine
❏ Vitals q4h
❏ Strict I/O
❏ Fortaz 2 g IV q8h
❏ Vancomycin 1 g IV q6h
❏ Claforan 1 g IV q12h
❏ Erythromycin 800 mg IV q6h

Identify the orders that require calculations.

Set up and solve each problem using dimensional analysis.

1. Calculate how many mEq/hr of KCl the patient will receive IV.

2. Calculate cc/hr to set the IV pump to infuse Fortaz 2 g. Supply: Fortaz 2-g vial to be reconstituted with 10 mL of sterile water and further diluted in 50 cc D5W to infuse over 30 min.

3. Calculate cc/hr to set the IV pump to infuse vancomycin 1 g. Supply: vancomycin 500-mg vial to be reconstituted with 10 mL of sterile water and further diluted in 100 cc of D5W to infuse over 60 min.

4. Calculate cc/hr to set the IV pump to infuse Claforan 1 g. Supply: Claforan 600 mg/4 mL to be further diluted with 100 cc D5W to infuse over 1 hr.

5. Calculate mL/hr to set the IV pump to infuse erythromycin 800 mg. Supply: Erythromycin 1-g vial to be diluted with 20 mL sterile water and further diluted in 250 mL of NS to infuse over 60 min.

■ CASE STUDY 8   Pneumonia

A patient is admitted to the hospital with fever, cough, chills, and dyspnea to rule out pneumonia. The orders from the physician include:

- ❏ IV 600 cc D5W q8h
- ❏ I/O
- ❏ Vitals q4h
- ❏ Complete blood count, electrolytes, chest x-ray, ABGs, sputum specimen, blood cultures, and bronchoscopy
- ❏ Bed rest
- ❏ Humidified O_2 at 4 L/min per nasal cannula
- ❏ High-calorie diet
- ❏ Encourage oral fluids of 2000 to 3000 mL/day
- ❏ Pulse oximetry qAM
- ❏ Clindamycin 400 mg IV q6h
- ❏ Albuterol respiratory treatments
- ❏ Guaifenesin 200 mg PO q4h
- ❏ Terbutaline 2.5 mg PO tid
- ❏ MS Contrin 30 mg PO q4h prn

Identify the orders that require calculations.

Set up and solve each problem using dimensional analysis.

1. Calculate cc/hr to set the IV pump to infuse clindamycin 400 mg. Supply: Clindamycin 600 mg/4 mL to be further diluted with 50 cc D5W to infuse over 1 hr.

2. Calculate gtt/min to infuse the clindamycin using macrotubing (20 gtt/mL).

3. Calculate how many cc of guaifenesin the patient will receive from a stock bottle labeled 30 mg/tsp.

4. Calculate how many tablets of terbutaline the patient will receive from a unit dose of 5 mg/tablet.

5. Calculate how many tablets of MS Contrin the patient will receive from a unit dose of 30 mg/tablet.

■ CASE STUDY 9   Pain

A patient is admitted to the hospital with intractable bone pain secondary to prostate cancer. The orders from the physician include:

❑ IV D5W/$\frac{1}{2}$ NS with 20 mEq KCl/L at 60 cc/hr
❑ IV 500 cc NS with 25 mg Dilaudid and 50 mg Thorazine at 21 cc/hr
❑ Heparin 25,000 units/250 cc D5W at 11 cc/hr
❑ Bed rest
❑ Do not resuscitate
❑ O_2 at 2 L/min per nasal cannula
❑ Bumex 2 mg IV qAM after albumin infusion
❑ Albumin 12.5 g IV qAM

Identify the orders that require calculations.

Set up and solve each problem using dimensional analysis.

1. Calculate how many mEq/hr of KCl the patient is receiving.

2. Calculate how many mg/hr of Dilaudid the patient is receiving.

3. Calculate how many mg/hr of Thorazine the patient is receiving.

4. Calculate how many units/hr of heparin the patient is receiving.

5. Calculate how many mL of Bumex the patient will receive from a stock dose of 0.25 mg/mL.

■ CASE STUDY 10   Cirrhosis

A patient is admitted to the hospital with ascites, stomach pain, dyspnea, and a history of cirrhosis of the liver. The orders from the physician include:

❑ IV D5W/$\frac{1}{2}$ NS with 20 mEq KCl at 125 cc/hr
❑ IV Zantac 150 mg/250 cc NS at 11 cc/hr
❑ O_2 at 2 L/min per nasal cannula
❑ Type and crossmatch for 2 units of packed red blood cells, complete blood count, liver panel, PT/PTT, SMA-12.
❑ Carafate 1 g q4h PO
❑ Vitamin K 10 mg SQ qAM
❑ Spironolactone 50 mg PO bid
❑ Lasix 80 mg IV qAM
❑ Measure abdominal girth qAM
❑ Sodium restriction to 500 mg/day
❑ Fluid restriction to 1500 cc/day

Identify the orders that require calculations.

Set up and solve each problem using dimensional analysis.

1. Calculate the gtt/min using macrotubing (20 gtt/mL).

2. Calculate the mg/hr of Zantac the patient is receiving.

3. Calculate how many mL of vitamin K the patient will receive SQ from a unit dose labeled 10 mg/mL.

4. Calculate how many tablets of spironolactone the patient will receive from a unit dose labeled 25 mg/tablet.

5. Calculate how many mL of Lasix the patient will receive from a unit dose labeled 10 mg/mL.

■ CASE STUDY 11   Hyperemesis Gravidarum

A 14-year-old patient is admitted to the hospital with weight loss and dehydration secondary to hyperemesis gravidarum. The orders from the physician include:

❑ Bed rest with bathroom privileges
❑ Obtain weight daily
❑ Vital q4h

❑ Test urine for ketones
❑ Urinalysis, complete blood count, electrolytes, liver enzymes, and bilirubin
❑ NPO for 48 hr, then advance diet to clear liquid, full liquid, and as tolerated
❑ IV D5 $\frac{1}{2}$ NS at 150 cc/hr for 8 hr, then decrease to 100 cc/hr
❑ Observe for signs of metabolic acidosis, jaundice, or hemorrhage
❑ Monitor intake and output
❑ Droperidol (Inapsine) 1 mg IV q4h prn for nausea
❑ Metoclopramide (Reglan) 20 mg IV in 50 mL of D5W to infuse over 15 min
❑ Diphenhydramine (Benadryl) 25 mg IV q3h prn for nausea
❑ Dexamethasone (Decadron) 4 mg IV q6h

Identify the orders that require calculations.

Set up and solve each problem using dimensional analysis.

1. Calculate gtt/min using macrotubing (20 gtt/mL) to infuse 150 cc/hr, then 100 cc/hr.

2. Calculate how many mL of droperidol the patient will receive IV. Supply: 2.5 mg/mL

3. Calculate mL/hr to set the IV pump to infuse metoclopramide (Reglan) 20 mg in 50 mL of D5W to infuse over 15 min.

4. Calculate how many mL of diphenhydramine (Benadryl) the patient will receive IV. Supply: 10 mg/mL.

5. Calculate how many mL of dexamethasone (Decadron) the patient will receive IV. Supply: 4 mg/mL.

■ **CASE STUDY 12**   **Preeclampsia**

A nulliparous female is admitted to the hospital with pregnancy-induced hypertension. The orders from the physician include:

❑ Complete bed rest in left lateral position
❑ Insert Foley catheter and check hourly for protein and specific gravity
❑ Daily weight
❑ Methyldopa (Aldomet) 250 mg PO tid
❑ Hydralazine (Apresoline) 5 mg IV every 20 min for blood pressure over 160/100

- ❏ Complete blood count, liver enzymes, chemistry panel, clotting studies, type and crossmatch, and urinalysis
- ❏ Magnesium sulfate 4 g in 250 mL D5LR loading dose to infuse over 30 min
- ❏ Magnesium sulfate 40 g in 1000 mL LR to infuse at 1 g/hr
- ❏ Keep calcium gluconate and intubation equipment at the bedside
- ❏ Nifedipine (Procardia) 10 mg sublingual for blood pressure over 160/100 and repeat in 15 min if needed.
- ❏ Keep lights dimmed and maintain a quiet environment
- ❏ Monitor blood pressure, pulse, and respiratory rate, fetal heart rate (FHR) contractions every 15 to 30 min, and deep tendon reflexes (DTR) hourly
- ❏ Monitor intake and output, proteinuria, presence of headache, visual disturbances, and epigastric pain hourly
- ❏ Restrict hourly fluid intake to 100 to 125 mL/hr

Identify the orders that require calculations.

Set up and solve each problem using dimensional analysis.

1. Calculate how many tablets of methyldopa (Aldomet) will be given PO. Supply: 500 mg/tablet.

2. Calculate how many mL of hydralazine (Apresoline) will be given IV. Supply: 20 mg/mL.

3. Calculate mL/hr to set the IV pump to infuse magnesium sulfate 4 g in 250 mL D5W loading dose to infuse over 30 min.

4. Calculate mL/hr to set the IV pump to infuse magnesium sulfate 40 g in 1000 mL LR to infuse at 1 g/hr.

5. Calculate how many capsules of nifedipine (Procardia) will be needed to give the sublingual dose. Supply: 10 mg/capsule.

■ CASE STUDY 13 Premature Labor

A 35-year-old female in the 30th week of gestation is admitted to the hospital in premature labor. The orders from the physician include:

- ❏ Bed rest in left lateral position
- ❏ Monitor intake and output
- ❏ Daily weights
- ❏ Continuous fetal monitoring

❏ Monitor blood pressure, pulse rate, respirations, fetal heart rate, uterine contraction pattern, and neurologic reflexes

❏ Keep calcium gluconate at the bedside

❏ Initiate magnesium sulfate 4 g in 250 cc LR loading dose over 20 min, then 2 g in 250 cc LR at 2 g/hr until contractions stop

❏ Continue tocolytic therapy with terbutaline (Brethine) 0.25 mg SQ every 30 min for 2 hr after contractions stop

❏ Give nifedipine (Procardia) 10 mg sublingual now, then 20 mg PO q6h after infusion of magnesium sulfate and contractions have stopped

❏ Betamethasone 12 mg IM × 2 doses 12 hr apart

❏ IV LR 1000 cc over 8 hr

Identify the orders that require calculations.

Set up and solve each problem using dimensional analysis.

1. Calculate cc/hr to set the IV pump to infuse the loading dose magnesium sulfate 4 g in 250 cc LR over 20 min and the 2 g/hr maintenance dose.

2. Calculate how many mL of terbutaline (Brethine) will be given SQ. Supply: 1 mg/mL.

3. Calculate how many capsules of nifedipine (Procardia) will be given PO q6h. Supply: 10 mg/capsule.

4. Betamethasone 12 mg IM × 2 doses 12 hr apart. Supply: 6 mg/mL.

5. Calculate cc/hr to set the IV pump to infuse LR 1000 cc over 8 hr.

■ CASE STUDY 14   Cystic Fibrosis

A 10-year-old child weighing 65 lb is admitted to the hospital with pulmonary exacerbation. The orders from the physician include:

❏ Complete blood count with differential, ABGs, chest x-ray, urinalysis, chemistry panel, and sputum culture

❏ IV 0.9% normal saline at 75 cc/hr

❏ Daily weights

❏ Monitor vitals q4h

❏ Oxygen at 2 L/min with pulse oximetry checks to maintain oxygen saturation above 92%

❏ Pancrease 2 capsules PO with meals and snacks

❏ High-calorie, high-protein diet

❏ Multivitamin 1 tablet PO daily

❑ Tagamet 30 mg/kg/day PO in four divided doses with meals and HS with a snack.

❑ Clindamycin 10 mg/kg IV q6h

❑ Postural drainage and percussion after aerosolized treatments

❑ Albuterol treatments with 2 inhalations q4h to 6h

❑ Terbutaline PO 2.5 mg q6h

❑ Tobramycin 1.5 mg/kg q6h

❑ Tobramycin peak and trough levels after fourth dose

Identify the orders that require calculations.

Set up and solve each problem using dimensional analysis.

1. Calculate gtt/min using macrotubing (15 gtt/mL).

2. Calculate how many tablets of Tagamet will be given PO with meals and HS snack. Supply: 200 mg/tablet.

3. Calculate how many mg of clindamycin the patient will receive, how many mL to draw from the vial, and mL/hr to set the IV pump. Supply: 150 mg/mL vial to be further diluted in 50 mL of NS and infused over 20 min.

4. Calculate how many tablets of terbutaline will be given PO. Supply: 2.5 mg/tablet.

5. Calculate how many mg of tobramycin the patient will receive, how many mL to draw from the vial, and cc/hr to set the IV pump. Supply: 40 mg/mL vial to be further diluted in 50 mL of NS and infused over 30 min.

■ CASE STUDY 15   Respiratory Syncytial Virus (RSV)

A 2-year-old child weighing 30 lb is admitted to the hospital for severe respiratory distress. The orders from the physician include:

❑ Complete blood count with differential, electrolytes, blood culture, chest x-ray, and nasal washing

❑ Humidified oxygen therapy to keep oxygen saturation >92%

❑ Continuous pulse oximetry

❑ IV D5W$\frac{1}{2}$ NS at 50 cc/hr

❑ Elevate HOB

❑ Vitals q2h

❑ Contact isolation

❏ Cardiorespiratory monitor
❏ Strict intake and output with urine specific gravities
❏ Acetaminophen elixir 120 mg q4h prn for temperature >101°F
❏ Aminophylline loading dose of 5 mg/kg to infuse over 30 min and maintenance dose of 0.8 mg/kg/hr
❏ Ribavirin (Virazole) inhalation therapy × 12 hr/day
❏ NPO with respiratory rate >60
❏ RespiGam 750 mg/kg IV monthly
❏ Pediapred 1.5 mg/kg/day in three divided doses
❏ Ampicillin 100 mg/kg/day in divided doses q6h

Identify the orders that require calculations.

Set up and solve each problem using dimensional analysis.

1. Calculate how many mL of acetaminophen elixir the patient will receive. Supply: 120 mg/5 mL.

2. Calculate how many mg of aminophylline the patient will receive and the cc/hr to set the IV pump for the loading dose, then calculate the cc/hr to set the IV pump for the maintenance dose. Supply: 250 mg/100 mL.

3. Calculate how many mg of RespiGam the patient will receive IV on a monthly infusion.

4. Calculate how many mL/dose of Pediapred the patient will receive. Supply: 15 mg/5 mL.

5. Calculate how many mg/dose of ampicillin the patient will receive IV, how many mL to draw from the vial, and cc/hr to set the IV pump. Supply: 1-g vials to be diluted with 10 mL of NS and further diluted in 50 cc NS to infuse over 30 min.

■ **CASE STUDY 16**   **Leukemia**

A 14-year-old child is admitted to the hospital with fever of unknown origin (FUO) after chemotherapy administration. The orders from the physician include:

❏ Complete blood count with differential, bone marrow aspiration, chemistry panel, PT/PTT, blood cultures, urinalysis, and type and crossmatch
❏ Regular diet as tolerated
❏ Vitals q4h
❏ Daily weights

❏ Monitor intake and output
❏ Type and cross for 2 units PRBCs
❏ Irradiate all blood products
❏ Infuse 6 pack of platelets for counts <20,000
❏ IV D5W/NS with 20 mEq KCl 1000 mL/8 hr
❏ Allopurinol 200 mg PO tid
❏ Fortaz 1 g IV q6h
❏ Aztreonam (Azactam) 2 g IV q12h
❏ Flagyl 500 mg IV q8h
❏ Acetaminophen two tablets q4h prn

Identify the orders that require calculations.

Set up and solve each problem using dimensional analysis.

1. Calculate mL/hr to set the IV pump.

2. Calculate how many tablets of allopurinol will be given PO.
   Supply: 100 mg/tablet.

3. Calculate how many mL/hr to set the IV pump to infuse Fortaz. Supply:
   1-g vial to be diluted with 10 mL of sterile water and further diluted in
   50 mL NS to infuse over 30 min.

4. Calculate how many mL of aztreonam to draw from the vial. Supply: 2-g
   vial to be diluted with 10 mL of sterile water and further diluted in
   100 mL NS to infuse over 60 min.

5. Calculate how many mL/hr to set the IV pump to infuse Flagyl. Supply:
   500 mg/100 mL to infuse over 1 hr.

■ CASE STUDY 17   Sepsis

A neonate born at 32 weeks' gestation (weight 2005 g) is admitted to the
Neonatal Intensive Care Unit (NICU) with a diagnosis of sepsis. The orders
from the physician include:

❏ Admit to NICU with continuous cardiorespiratory monitoring
❏ Complete blood counts, blood and urine cultures, chest x-ray, bilirubin,
   ABGs, theophylline levels, and lumbar puncture
❏ Strict intake and output
❏ Daily weight
❏ Vitals q3h
❏ NG breast milk diluted with sterile water 120 cc/day with feedings q3h

❏ IV D10 and 20% lipids 120 cc/kg/day
❏ Aminophylline 5 mg/kg IV q6h
❏ Cefotaxime (Claforan) 50 mg/kg q12h
❏ Vancomycin 10 mg/kg/dose q12h

Identify the orders that require calculations.

Set up and solve each problem using dimensional analysis.

1. Calculate how many cc the child will receive with every feeding.

2. Calculate how many mL/hr the child will receive IV.

3. Calculate how many mg of aminophylline the child will receive q6h. Calculate how many mL/hr you will set the IV pump. Supply: 50 mg/10 mL to infuse over 5 min.

4. Calculate how many mg of cefotaxime the child will receive every 12 hr. Calculate how many mL/hr you will set the IV pump. Supply: 40 mg/mL to infuse over 30 min.

5. Calculate how many mg of vancomycin the child will receive every 12 hr. Calculate how many mL/hr you will set the IV pump. Supply: 5 mg/mL to infuse over 1 hr.

■ **CASE STUDY 18**   **Bronchopulmonary Dysplasia**

A neonate born at 24 weeks' gestation diagnosed with respiratory distress syndrome and respiratory failure is now 28 weeks' gestation (weight 996 g) with bronchopulmonary dysplasia. This child remains in the Neonatal Intensive Care Unit (NICU) on oxygen therapy and enteral feedings. The orders from the physician include:

❏ Complete blood count, chemistry panel, ABGs, chest x-ray, CPPD with nebulizations, glucose monitoring, caffeine citrate levels, and newborn screen
❏ NG feedings with Special Care with Iron 120 kcal/kg/day
❏ Chlorothiazide (Diuril) 10 mg/kg/day PO
❏ Fer-In-Sol 2 mg/kg/day
❏ Vitamin E 25 units/kg/day in divided doses q12h
❏ Caffeine citrate 5 mg/kg/dose daily

Identify the orders that require calculations.

Set up and solve each problem using dimensional analysis.

1. Calculate how many total calories the child will receive daily. Calculate how many cc/day the child will receive. Supply: 24 kcal/oz.

2. Calculate how many mg of chlorothiazide the child will receive daily. Calculate how many mL/day the child will receive. Supply: 250 mg/5 mL.

3. Calculate how many mg of Fer-In-Sol the child will receive daily. Calculate how many mL/day the child will receive. Supply: 15 mg/0.6 mL.

4. Calculate how many units/dose of vitamin E the child will receive every 12 hr. Calculate how many mL/dose the child will receive. Supply: 67 units/mL.

5. Calculate how many mg of caffeine citrate the child will receive daily. Calculate how many mL/dose the child will receive. Supply: 10 mg/mL.

■ CASE STUDY 19   Cerebral Palsy

A 13-year-old child (weight 38 kg) with cerebral palsy being cared for in a children's facility is admitted to the hospital for seizure evaluation. The orders from the physician include:

❑ Complete blood count, chemistry panel, urinalysis, dilantin levels, EEG, and CT scan
❑ Vitals q4h
❑ Seizure precautions
❑ Lactulose 3 g PO tid
❑ Valproic acid (Depakote) 30 mg/kg/day PO in three divided doses
❑ Diazepam (Valium) 2.5 mg PO daily
❑ Chlorothiazide (Thiazide) 250 mg PO daily
❑ Phenytoin (Dilantin) 5 mg/kg/day PO in three divided doses

Identify the orders that require calculations.

Set up and solve each problem using dimensional analysis.

1. Calculate how many mL of lactulose the child will receive. Supply: 10 g/15 mL.

2. Calculate how many tablets of Depakote the child will receive per dose. Supply: 125 mg/tablet.

3. Calculate how many tablets of diazepam the child will receive per dose. Supply: 5 mg/tablet.

4. Calculate how many tablets of chlorothiazide the child will receive per dose. Supply: 250 mg/tablet.

5. Calculate how many mL of Dilantin the child will receive per dose. Supply: 125 mg/5 mL.

■ CASE STUDY 20   Hyperbilirubinemia

A 4-day-old neonate born at 35 weeks' gestation (weight 2210 g) is readmitted to the hospital for treatment of dehydration and jaundice with a bilirubin level of 21 mg/dL. The orders from the physician include:

❏ Phototherapy and exchange transfusion through an umbilical venous catheter
❏ Total and indirect bilirubin levels, electrolytes, complete blood count, and type and crossmatch
❏ Continuous cardiorespiratory monitoring
❏ Vitals q2h
❏ Monitor intake and output
❏ Albumin 5% infusion 1 g/kg 1 hr before exchange
❏ Ampicillin 100 mg/kg/dose IV q12h
❏ Gentamicin 4 mg/kg/dose IV q12h
❏ NPO before exchange, then 120 cc/kg/day formula
❏ IV D10W 120 cc/kg/day

Identify the orders that require calculations.

Set up and solve each problem using dimensional analysis.

1. Calculate how many g of albumin the infant will receive before exchange therapy.

2. Calculate how many mg/dose of ampicillin the infant will receive every 12 hr. Calculate how many mL the infant will receive. Supply: 250 mg/5 mL IV push over 5 min.

3. Calculate how many mg/dose of gentamicin the infant will receive every 12 hr. Calculate how many mL the infant will receive. Supply: 2 mg/mL.

4. Calculate how many cc/day of formula the infant will receive.

5. Calculate how many cc/hr to set the IV pump.

■ CASE STUDY 21 | Spontaneous Abortion

A 31-year-old female is admitted to the hospital to control severe hemorrhage after a spontaneous abortion. The orders from the physician include:

❏ CBC to determine blood loss
❏ WBC with differential to rule out infection
❏ Type and crossmatch for 2 units of blood
❏ Obtain Coombs' test to determine Rh status
❏ Administer Rhogam 300 mcg IM if patient is Rh-negative with a negative indirect Coombs' test
❏ IV D5/0.9% NS at 100 cc/hr
❏ IV oxytocin (Pitocin) 10 Units infused at 20 mU/min
❏ Prepare for a dilatation and curettage (D&C)
❏ Complete bed rest. Monitor bedpan for contents for intrauterine material
❏ Administer meperidine (Demerol) 50 mg IM q4h for severe discomfort
❏ Administer ibuprofen 400 mg PO q6h for mild discomfort
❏ Monitor vital signs q4h for 24 hr
❏ Monitor urine output
❏ Note the amount, color, and odor of vaginal bleeding

Identify the orders that require calculations.

Set up and solve each problem using dimensional analysis.

1. Calculate how many mL of Rhogam the patient will receive.
   Supply: Rhogam 300 mcg/mL vial. Administer into the deltoid muscle within 72 hr of abortion.

2. Calculate gtt/min using macrotubing (15 gtt/mL).

3. Calculate how many cc/hr to set the IV pump to infuse oxytocin 10 units.
   Supply: Oxytocin 10 units in 500 mL D5/NS.

4. Calculate how many mL of meperidine (Demerol) will be given IM. The prefilled syringe is labeled 100 mg/mL.

5. Calculate how many tablets of ibuprofen will be given PO.
   Supply: 200 mg/tablet.

■ **CASE STUDY 22**   **Bipolar Disorder**

A 25-year-old female is brought to the hospital by her friends after she fainted at the PowerShop. Her friends reported that she has been very sad, withdrawn, and not involved in any of her usual activities for some time but had suddenly become "full of energy" at the PowerShop. The orders from the physician include:

❏ CBC and electrolytes
❏ WBC with differential
❏ BUN and creatinine
❏ Liver panel
❏ Lithium levels
❏ IV 0.9% NS at 75 cc/hr
❏ Lithium 300 mg PO tid
❏ Clonazepam 0.5 mg PO bid; increase to 1 mg PO bid after 3 days
❏ Doxepin 50 mg PO tid
❏ Intake and output

Identify the orders that require calculations.

Set up and solve each problem using dimensional analysis.

1. Calculate the gtt/min using macrotubing (20 gtt/mL).

2. Calculate how many capsules of lithium will be given PO. Supply: 150 mg/capsule.

3. Calculate how many tablets of clonazepam will be given PO. Supply: 0.5-mg tablets.

4. Calculate how many tablets of clonazepam will be given PO after 3 days. Supply: 0.5-mg tablets.

5. Calculate how many tablets of doxepin will be given PO. Supply: 25-mg tablets.

■ **CASE STUDY 23**   **Anorexia Nervosa**

A 17-year-old female high school student is admitted by her parents for self-induced starvation, vomiting, and laxative abuse. The 12-week hospital stay is for management of diet with a 1- to 2-lb/week weight gain goal. The orders from the physician include:

❏ DSM-IV evaluation
❏ Nutritional consult for 1500-calorie diet advance to 3500 calories over 12 weeks
❏ CBC, platelet count, and sedimentation rate
❏ WBC with differential
❏ Electrolytes, BUN, and creatinine
❏ Liver enzymes

❏ Urinalysis
❏ ECG
❏ Daily weight
❏ Intake and output
❏ 1000 cc IV D5/LR with 20 mEq K+ to infuse over 8 hr
❏ Olanzapine (Zyprexa) 10 mg PO HS
❏ Fluoxetine (Prozac) 60 mg/day PO qAM
❏ Amitriptyline 25 mg PO qid
❏ Cyproheptadine 32 mg/day PO in 4 divided doses

Identify the orders that require calculations.

Set up and solve each problem using dimensional analysis.

1. Calculate how many cc/hr to set the IV pump.

2. Calculate how many tablets of olanzapine (Zyprexa) will be given at HS.
   Supply: 5-mg tablets.

3. Calculate how many mL of fluoxetine (Prozac) will be given PO.
   Supply: 20 mg/5 mL.

4. Calculate how many tablets of amitriptyline will be given PO.
   Supply: 10 mg/5 mL.

5. Calculate how many mL of cyproheptadine will be given PO.
   Supply: 2 mg/5 mL.

■ CASE STUDY 24   Clinical Depression

A 44-year-old successful businessman with a wife and two children, and diagnosed with clinical depression, has received several months of treatment with antidepressants and psychotherapy. The depression has not responded to therapy. He has become suicidal, and he has agreed to try electroconvulsive therapy (also called ECT). The orders from the physician include:

❏ Admit for ECT
❏ CBC and urinalysis
❏ ECG
❏ NPO after midnight
❏ Obtain AM weight
❏ Obtain baseline vitals 60 min before procedure
❏ Start IV D5/0.45% at 100 mL/hr
❏ Administer glycopyrrolate (Robinul) 4.4 mcg/kg IM 30 min
   preoperatively
❏ Zoloft 50 mg PO qAM
❏ Sinequan 25 mg PO tid
❏ Parnate 30 mg/day PO in 2 divided doses

Identify the orders that require calculations.

Set up and solve each problem using dimensional analysis.

1. Calculate the gtt/min using macrotubing (10 gtt/mL).

2. Calculate how many mL of glycopyrrolate (Robinul) will be given IM. Supply: 200 mcg/mL. Patient weight: 175 lb.

3. Calculate how many tablets of sertraline (Zoloft) will be given PO. Supply: 50-mg tablets.

4. Calculate how many capsules of doxepin (Sinequan) will be given PO. Supply: 25-mg capsules.

5. Calculate how many tablets of tranylcypromine (Parnate) will be given PO. Supply: 10-mg tablets.

■ CASE STUDY 25   Alzheimer's Disease

A 62-year-old executive is experiencing difficulty remembering and performing familiar tasks, problems with abstract thinking, and changes in mood and behavior. He is hospitalized for evaluation. The orders from the physician include:

- ❏ CT of the brain
- ❏ EEG and cerebral blood flow studies
- ❏ CBC and electrolytes
- ❏ Cerebrospinal fluid analysis
- ❏ Urinalysis
- ❏ 1000 mL IV D5/0.45% NS to infuse over 8 hr
- ❏ Donepezil (Aricept) 5 mg PO HS
- ❏ Thioridazine (Mellaril) 25 mg PO tid
- ❏ Imipramine (Tofranil) 50 mg PO qid
- ❏ Temazepam (Restoril) 7.5 mg PO HS

Identify the orders that require calculations.

Set up and solve each problem using dimensional analysis.

1. Calculate gtt/min using macrotubing (15 gtt/mL).

2. Calculate how many tablets of donepezil (Aricept) will be given PO. Supply: 5-mg tablets.

3. Calculate how many tablets of thioridazine (Mellaril) will be given PO. Supply: 25-mg tablets.

4. Calculate how many tablets of imipramine (Tofranil) will be given PO. Supply: 25-mg tablets.

5. Calculate how many tablets of temazepam (Restoril) will be given PO. Supply: 15-mg tablets.

ANSWER KEY FOR SECTION 3: CASE STUDIES

Case Study 1: **Congestive Heart Failure**

Orders requiring calculations: IV of D5W/$\frac{1}{2}$ NS at 50 cc/hr; weight gain; furosemide 40 mg IV qd; digoxin 0.125 mg PO qd; KCl 20 mEq PO tid

1. $\dfrac{50 \text{ cc}}{\text{hr}} \left| \dfrac{60 \text{ gtt}}{\text{mL}} \right| \dfrac{1 \text{ hr}}{60 \text{ min}} \left| \dfrac{50 \times 1}{60} = \dfrac{50 \text{ gtt}}{\text{min}}\right.$

2. $\dfrac{10 \text{ lb}}{} \left| \dfrac{1 \text{ kg}}{2.2 \text{ lb}} \right| \dfrac{10 \times 1}{2.2} \left| \dfrac{10}{2.2} = 4.5 \text{ kg}\right.$

3. $\dfrac{40 \text{ mg}}{} \left| \dfrac{\text{mL}}{10 \text{ mg}} \right| \dfrac{4}{1} = 4 \text{ mL}$

4. $\dfrac{0.125 \text{ mg}}{} \left| \dfrac{\text{tablet}}{0.25 \text{ mg}} \right| \dfrac{0.125}{0.25} = 0.5 \text{ tablet}$

5. $\dfrac{20 \text{ mEq}}{} \left| \dfrac{\text{tablet}}{10 \text{ mEq}} \right| \dfrac{2}{1} = 2 \text{ tablets}$

Case Study 2: **Congestive COPD/Emphysema**

Orders requiring calculations: IV of D5W/$\frac{1}{2}$ NS 1000 cc/8 hr; aminophylline IV loading dose of 5.6 mg/kg over 30 min followed by 0.5 mg/kg/hr continuous IV; erythromycin 800 mg IV q6h; accurate I/O.

1. $\dfrac{1000 \text{ cc}}{8 \text{ hr}} \left| \dfrac{1000}{8} = \dfrac{125 \text{ cc}}{\text{hr}}\right.$

2. $\dfrac{5.6 \text{ mg}}{\text{kg}/30 \text{ min}} \left| \dfrac{100 \text{ cc}}{100 \text{ mg}} \right| \dfrac{1 \text{ kg}}{2.2 \text{ lb}} \left| \dfrac{140 \text{ lb}}{} \right| \dfrac{60 \text{ min}}{1 \text{ hr}} \left| \dfrac{5.6 \times 14 \times 6}{3 \times 2.2}\right.$

$\dfrac{470.4}{6.6} = \dfrac{71.3 \text{ cc}}{\text{hr}} \text{ or } \dfrac{71 \text{ cc}}{\text{hr}}$

3. $\dfrac{0.5 \text{ mg}}{\text{kg}/\text{hr}} \left| \dfrac{250 \text{ cc}}{1 \text{ g}} \right| \dfrac{1 \text{ g}}{1000 \text{ mg}} \left| \dfrac{1 \text{ kg}}{2.2 \text{ lb}} \right| \dfrac{140 \text{ lb}}{} \left| \dfrac{0.5 \times 25 \times 1 \times 14}{10 \times 2.2}\right.$

$\dfrac{175}{22} = \dfrac{7.9 \text{ cc}}{\text{hr}} \text{ or } \dfrac{8 \text{ cc}}{\text{hr}}$

4. $\dfrac{800 \text{ mg}}{} \left| \dfrac{20 \text{ mL}}{1 \text{ g}} \right| \dfrac{1 \text{ g}}{1000 \text{ mg}} \left| \dfrac{8 \times 2}{1} = 16 \text{ mL}\right.$

$\dfrac{266 \text{ cc}}{1 \text{ hr}} = \dfrac{266 \text{ cc}}{\text{hr}}$

5. $\dfrac{3 \text{ L}}{\text{day}} \left| \dfrac{\text{day}}{3 \text{ shifts}} \right| \dfrac{1000 \text{ mL}}{1 \text{ L}} \left| \dfrac{1000}{1} = \dfrac{1000 \text{ mL}}{\text{shift}}\right.$

Case Study 3: **Small Cell Lung Cancer**

Orders requiring calculations: IV D5W/$\frac{1}{2}$ NS 1000 cc with 10 mEq KCl at 125 cc/hr; Neupogen 5 mcg/kg SQ daily; gentamicin 80 mg IV q8h; Decadron 8 mg IV daily; Fortaz 1 g IV q8h

1. $\dfrac{125 \text{ cc}}{\text{hr}} \left| \dfrac{20 \text{ gtt}}{\text{mL}} \right| \dfrac{1 \text{ hr}}{60 \text{ min}} \left| \dfrac{125 \times 2 \times 1}{6} \right| \dfrac{250}{6} = \dfrac{41.6 \text{ or } 42 \text{ gtt}}{\text{min}}$

2. $\dfrac{5 \text{ mcg}}{\text{kg}} \left| \dfrac{1 \text{ kg}}{2.2 \text{ lb}} \right| \dfrac{160 \text{ lb}}{} \left| \dfrac{5 \times 1 \times 160}{2.2} \right| \dfrac{800}{2.2} = 363.6 \text{ mcg or } 364 \text{ mcg}$

3. $\dfrac{80 \text{ mg}}{} \left| \dfrac{\text{mL}}{40 \text{ mg}} \right| \dfrac{8}{4} = 2 \text{ mL}$

$\dfrac{102 \text{ cc}}{1 \text{ hr}} = \dfrac{102 \text{ cc}}{\text{hr}}$

4. $\dfrac{8 \text{ mg}}{} \left| \dfrac{\text{mL}}{4 \text{ mg}} \right| \dfrac{8}{4} = 2 \text{ mL}$

5. $\dfrac{50 \text{ mL}}{30 \text{ min}} \left| \dfrac{60 \text{ min}}{1 \text{ hr}} \right| \dfrac{50 \times 6}{3 \times 1} \left| \dfrac{300}{3} = \dfrac{100 \text{ mL}}{\text{hr}}\right.$

Case Study 4: Acquired Immunodeficiency Syndrome (AIDS)

Orders requiring calculations: IV D5W/$\frac{1}{2}$ NS at 150 cc/hr; acyclovir 350 mg IV q8h; Neupogen 300 mcg SQ daily; Epogen 100 units/kg SQ three times a week; vancomycin 800 mg IV q6h

1.
$$\frac{150 \text{ cc}}{\text{hr}} \Big| \frac{20 \text{ gtt}}{\text{mL}} \Big| \frac{1 \text{ hr}}{60 \text{ min}} \Big| \frac{150 \times 2 \times 1}{6} \Big| \frac{300}{6} = \frac{50 \text{ gtt}}{\text{min}}$$

2.
$$\frac{350 \text{ mg}}{} \Big| \frac{10 \text{ mL}}{500 \text{ mg}} \Big| \frac{35 \times 1}{5} \Big| \frac{35}{5} = 7 \text{ mL}$$

$$\frac{107 \text{ cc}}{1 \text{ hr}} \Big| \frac{107}{1} = \frac{107 \text{ cc}}{\text{hr}}$$

3.
$$\frac{300 \text{ mcg}}{} \Big| \frac{1 \text{ mL}}{300 \text{ mcg}} = 1 \text{ mL}$$

4.
$$\frac{100 \text{ units}}{\text{kg}} \Big| \frac{\text{mL}}{4000 \text{ units}} \Big| \frac{1 \text{ kg}}{2.2 \text{ lb}} \Big| \frac{100 \text{ lb}}{} \Big| \frac{10 \times 1 \times 1}{4 \times 2.2} \Big| \frac{10}{8.8} = 1.1 \text{ mL or 1 mL}$$

5.
$$\frac{800 \text{ mg}}{} \Big| \frac{10 \text{ mL}}{1 \text{ g}} \Big| \frac{1 \text{ g}}{1000 \text{ mg}} \Big| \frac{80 \times 1}{10} \Big| \frac{80}{10} = 8 \text{ mL}$$

$$\frac{108 \text{ mL}}{60 \text{ min}} \Big| \frac{60 \text{ min}}{1 \text{ hr}} \Big| \frac{108}{1} = \frac{108 \text{ cc}}{\text{hr}}$$

Case Study 5: Sickle Cell Anemia

Orders requiring calculations: IV D5W/$\frac{1}{2}$ NS at 150 cc/hr; Zofran 8 mg IV q8h; morphine sulfate 5 mg IV prn; Hydrea 10 mg/kg/day PO; folic acid 0.5 mg daily PO

1.
$$\frac{150 \text{ cc}}{\text{hr}} \Big| \frac{10 \text{ gtt}}{\text{mL}} \Big| \frac{1 \text{ hr}}{60 \text{ min}} \Big| \frac{150 \times 1 \times 1}{6} \Big| \frac{150}{6} = \frac{25 \text{ gtt}}{\text{min}}$$

2.
$$\frac{50 \text{ cc}}{15 \text{ min}} \Big| \frac{60 \text{ min}}{1 \text{ hr}} \Big| \frac{50 \times 60}{15 \times 1} \Big| \frac{3000}{15} = \frac{200 \text{ cc}}{\text{hr}}$$

3.
$$\frac{5 \text{ mg}}{} \Big| \frac{\text{mL}}{10 \text{ mg}} \Big| \frac{5}{10} = 0.5 \text{ mL}$$

4.
$$\frac{10 \text{ mg}}{\text{kg/day}} \Big| \frac{1 \text{ kg}}{2.2 \text{ lb}} \Big| \frac{125 \text{ lb}}{} \Big| \frac{10 \times 1 \times 125}{2.2} \Big| \frac{1250}{2.2} = \frac{568 \text{ mg}}{\text{day}}$$

5.
$$\frac{0.5 \text{ mg}}{} \Big| \frac{\text{tablet}}{1 \text{ mg}} \Big| \frac{0.5}{1} = 0.5 \text{ tablet}$$

Case Study 6: Deep Vein Thrombosis

Orders requiring calculations: IV D5W/$\frac{1}{2}$ NS with 20 mEq KCl at 50 cc/hr; heparin 5000 units IV push followed by continuous IV infusion of 1000 units/hr; Lasix 20 mg IV bid; morphine 5 mg IV q4h

1.
$$\frac{50 \text{ cc}}{\text{hr}} \Big| \frac{60 \text{ gtt}}{\text{mL}} \Big| \frac{1 \text{ hr}}{60 \text{ min}} \Big| \frac{50 \times 1}{} \Big| \frac{50}{} = \frac{50 \text{ gtt}}{\text{min}}$$

2.
$$\frac{5000 \text{ units}}{} \Big| \frac{\text{mL}}{10,000 \text{ units}} \Big| \frac{5}{10} = 0.5 \text{ mL}$$

3.
$$\frac{1000 \text{ units}}{\text{hr}} \Big| \frac{250 \text{ mL}}{25,000 \text{ units}} \Big| \frac{10}{} = \frac{10 \text{ mL}}{\text{hr}}$$

4.
$$\frac{20 \text{ mg}}{} \Big| \frac{\text{mL}}{10 \text{ mg}} \Big| \frac{2}{1} = 2 \text{ mL}$$

5.
$$\frac{5 \text{ mg}}{} \Big| \frac{\text{mL}}{10 \text{ mg}} \Big| \frac{5}{10} = 0.5 \text{ mL}$$

Case Study 7: Bone Marrow Transplant

Orders requiring calculations: IV D5W/$\frac{1}{2}$ NS with 20 mEq KCl/L at 80 cc/hr; Fortaz 2 g IV q8h; vancomycin 1 g IV q6h; Claforan 1 g IV q12h; erythromycin 800 mg IV q6h

1.
$$\frac{80 \text{ cc}}{\text{hr}} \Big| \frac{20 \text{ mEq}}{1 \text{ L}} \Big| \frac{1 \text{ L}}{1000 \text{ mL}} \Big| \frac{8 \times 2}{10} \Big| \frac{16}{10} = \frac{1.6 \text{ mEq}}{\text{hr}}$$

2. $\dfrac{\cancel{2\ \text{g}} \quad | \quad 10\ \boxed{\text{mL}} \quad | \quad 10}{\qquad\qquad | \quad \cancel{2\ \text{g}} \qquad} = 10\ \text{mL}$

$\dfrac{60\ \boxed{\text{cc}} \quad | \quad \cancel{60\ \text{min}} \quad | \quad 60 \times 6 \quad | \quad 360}{30\ \cancel{\text{min}} \quad | \quad 1\ \boxed{\text{hr}} \quad | \quad 3 \times 1 \quad | \quad 3} = 120\ \dfrac{\text{cc}}{\text{hr}}$

3. $\dfrac{\cancel{1\ \text{g}} \quad | \quad 10\ \boxed{\text{mL}} \quad | \quad 1000\ \cancel{\text{mg}} \quad | \quad 10 \times 10 \quad | \quad 100}{\qquad | \quad 500\ \text{mg} \quad | \quad \cancel{1\ \text{g}} \quad | \quad 5 \quad | \quad 5} = 20\ \text{mL}$

$\dfrac{120\ \boxed{\text{cc}} \quad | \quad \cancel{60\ \text{min}} \quad | \quad 120}{\cancel{60\ \text{min}} \quad | \quad 1\ \boxed{\text{hr}} \quad | \quad 1} = 120\ \dfrac{\text{cc}}{\text{hr}}$

4. $\dfrac{\cancel{1\ \text{g}} \quad | \quad 4\ \boxed{\text{mL}} \quad | \quad 1000\ \cancel{\text{mg}} \quad | \quad 4 \times 10 \quad | \quad 40}{\qquad | \quad 600\ \text{mg} \quad | \quad \cancel{1\ \text{g}} \quad | \quad 6 \quad | \quad 6} = 6.7\ \text{mL or } 7\ \text{mL}$

$\dfrac{107\ \boxed{\text{cc}} \quad | \quad 107}{1\ \boxed{\text{hr}} \quad | \quad 1} = 107\ \dfrac{\text{cc}}{\text{hr}}$

5. $\dfrac{800\ \text{mg} \quad | \quad 20\ \boxed{\text{mL}} \quad | \quad \cancel{1\ \text{g}} \quad | \quad 8 \times 2 \quad | \quad 16}{\qquad | \quad \cancel{1\ \text{g}} \quad | \quad 1000\ \text{mg} \quad | \quad 1 \quad | \quad 1} = 16\ \text{mL}$

$\dfrac{266\ \boxed{\text{mL}} \quad | \quad \cancel{60\ \text{min}} \quad | \quad 266}{\cancel{60\ \text{min}} \quad | \quad 1\ \boxed{\text{hr}} \quad | \quad 1} = 266\ \dfrac{\text{mL}}{\text{hr}}$

Case Study 8: **Pneumonia**

Orders requiring calculations: Clindamycin 400 mg IV q6h; guaifenesin 200 mg PO q4h; terbutaline 2.5 mg PO tid; MS Contin 30 mg PO q4h prn

1. $\dfrac{400\ \cancel{\text{mg}} \quad | \quad 4\ \boxed{\text{mL}} \quad | \quad 4 \times 4 \quad | \quad 16}{\qquad | \quad 600\ \cancel{\text{mg}} \quad | \quad 6 \quad | \quad 6} = 2.7\ \text{mL or } 3\ \text{mL}$

$\dfrac{53\ \boxed{\text{cc}} \quad | \quad 53}{\boxed{\text{hr}} \quad |} = 53\ \dfrac{\text{cc}}{\text{hr}}$

2. $\dfrac{53\ \cancel{\text{cc}} \quad | \quad 20\ \boxed{\text{gtt}} \quad | \quad 1\ \cancel{\text{hr}} \quad | \quad 53 \times 2 \times 1 \quad | \quad 106}{\cancel{\text{hr}} \quad | \quad \cancel{\text{mL}} \quad | \quad 60\ \boxed{\text{min}} \quad | \quad 6 \quad | \quad 6} = 18\ \dfrac{\text{gtt}}{\text{min}}$

3. $\dfrac{200\ \cancel{\text{mg}} \quad | \quad \cancel{\text{tsp}} \quad | \quad 5\ \boxed{\text{cc}} \quad | \quad 20 \times 5 \quad | \quad 100}{30\ \cancel{\text{mg}} \quad | \quad 1\ \cancel{\text{tsp}} \quad | \quad 3 \times 1 \quad | \quad 3} = 33\ \text{cc}$

4. $\dfrac{2.5\ \cancel{\text{mg}} \quad | \quad \boxed{\text{tablet}} \quad | \quad 2.5}{\qquad | \quad 5\ \cancel{\text{mg}} \quad | \quad 5} = 0.5\ \text{tablet}$

5. $\dfrac{30\ \cancel{\text{mg}} \quad | \quad \boxed{\text{tablet}} \quad | \quad 30}{30\ \cancel{\text{mg}} \quad | \quad 30} = 1\ \text{tablet}$

Case Study 9: **Pain**

Orders requiring calculations: IV D5W/$\frac{1}{2}$ NS with 20 mEq KCl/L at 60 cc/hr; IV 500 cc NS with 25 mg dilaudid and 50 mg thorazine at 21 cc/hr; Bumex 2 mg IV qAM after albumin infusion

1. $\dfrac{60\ \cancel{\text{cc}} \quad | \quad 20\ \boxed{\text{mEq}} \quad | \quad \cancel{1\ \text{L}} \quad | \quad 6 \times 2 \quad | \quad 12}{\boxed{\text{hr}} \quad | \quad \cancel{1\ \text{L}} \quad | \quad 1000\ \text{mL} \quad | \quad 10 \quad | \quad 10} = 1.2\ \dfrac{\text{mEq}}{\text{hr}}$

2. $\dfrac{21\ \cancel{\text{cc}} \quad | \quad 25\ \boxed{\text{mg}} \quad | \quad 21 \times 25 \quad | \quad 525}{\boxed{\text{hr}} \quad | \quad 500\ \cancel{\text{cc}} \quad | \quad 500 \quad | \quad 500} = 1.05\ \dfrac{\text{mg}}{\text{hr}}$

3. $\dfrac{21\ \cancel{\text{cc}} \quad | \quad 50\ \boxed{\text{mg}} \quad | \quad 21 \times 5 \quad | \quad 105}{\boxed{\text{hr}} \quad | \quad 500\ \cancel{\text{cc}} \quad | \quad 50 \quad | \quad 50} = 2.1\ \dfrac{\text{mg}}{\text{hr}}$

4. $\dfrac{11\ \cancel{\text{cc}} \quad | \quad 25,000\ \boxed{\text{units}} \quad | \quad 11 \times 2500 \quad | \quad 27,500}{\boxed{\text{hr}} \quad | \quad 250\ \cancel{\text{cc}} \quad | \quad 25 \quad | \quad 25} = 1100\ \dfrac{\text{units}}{\text{hr}}$

5. $\dfrac{2\ \cancel{\text{mg}} \quad | \quad \boxed{\text{mL}} \quad | \quad 2}{\qquad | \quad 0.25\ \cancel{\text{mg}} \quad | \quad 0.25} = 8\ \text{mL}$

Case Study 10: **Cirrhosis**

Orders requiring calculations: IV D5W/$\frac{1}{2}$ NS with 20 mEq KCl at 125 cc/hr; IV Zantac 150 mg/250 cc NS at 11 cc/hr; vitamin K 10 mg SQ qAM; Spironolactone 50 mg PO bid; Lasix 80 mg IV qAM

1. $\dfrac{125\ \cancel{\text{cc}} \quad | \quad 20\ \boxed{\text{gtt}} \quad | \quad 1\ \cancel{\text{hr}} \quad | \quad 125 \times 2 \times 1 \quad | \quad 250}{\cancel{\text{hr}} \quad | \quad \cancel{\text{mL}} \quad | \quad 60\ \boxed{\text{min}} \quad | \quad 6 \quad | \quad 6} = 41.66\ \text{or } 42\ \dfrac{\text{gtt}}{\text{min}}$

2. $\dfrac{11 \text{ cc}}{\text{hr}} \left| \dfrac{15\theta \text{ mg}}{25\theta \text{ cc}} \right| \dfrac{11 \times 15}{25} \left| \dfrac{165}{25} \right. = 6.6 \dfrac{\text{mg}}{\text{hr}}$

3. $\dfrac{10 \text{ mg}}{} \left| \dfrac{\text{mL}}{10 \text{ mg}} \right| \dfrac{10}{10} = 1 \text{ mL}$

4. $\dfrac{50 \text{ mg}}{} \left| \dfrac{\text{tablet}}{25 \text{ mg}} \right| \dfrac{50}{25} = 2 \text{ tablets}$

5. $\dfrac{8\theta \text{ mg}}{} \left| \dfrac{\text{mL}}{1\theta \text{ mg}} \right| \dfrac{8}{1} = 8 \text{ mL}$

Case Study 11: **Hyperemesis Gravidarum**

Orders requiring calculations: IV D5$\frac{1}{2}$ NS at 150 cc/hr and 100 cc/hr; droperidol (Inapsine) 1 mg IV; metoclopramide (Reglan) 20 mg IV in 50 mL of D5W to infuse over 15 min; diphenhydramine (Benadryl) 25 mg; dexamethasone (Decadron) 4 mg IV

1. $\dfrac{150 \text{ cc}}{\text{hr}} \left| \dfrac{2\theta \text{ gtt}}{\text{mL}} \right| \dfrac{1 \text{ hr}}{6\theta \text{ min}} \left| \dfrac{150 \times 2 \times 1}{6} \right| \dfrac{300}{6} = 50 \dfrac{\text{gtt}}{\text{min}}$

$\dfrac{100 \text{ cc}}{\text{hr}} \left| \dfrac{2\theta \text{ gtt}}{\text{mL}} \right| \dfrac{1 \text{ hr}}{6\theta \text{ min}} \left| \dfrac{100 \times 2 \times 1}{6} \right| \dfrac{200}{6} = 33.3 \text{ or } 33 \dfrac{\text{gtt}}{\text{min}}$

2. $\dfrac{1 \text{ mg}}{} \left| \dfrac{\text{mL}}{2.5 \text{ mg}} \right| \dfrac{1}{2.5} = 0.4 \text{ mL}$

3. $\dfrac{50 \text{ mL}}{15 \text{ min}} \left| \dfrac{60 \text{ min}}{1 \text{ hr}} \right| \dfrac{50 \times 60}{15 \times 1} \left| \dfrac{3000}{15} \right. = 200 \dfrac{\text{mL}}{\text{hr}}$

4. $\dfrac{25 \text{ mg}}{} \left| \dfrac{\text{mL}}{10 \text{ mg}} \right| \dfrac{25}{10} = 2.5 \text{ mL}$

5. $\dfrac{4 \text{ mg}}{} \left| \dfrac{\text{mL}}{4 \text{ mg}} \right| \dfrac{4}{4} = 1 \text{ mL}$

Case Study 12: **Preeclampsia**

Orders requiring calculations: Methyldopa (Aldomet) 250 mg; Hydralazine (Apresoline) 5 mg IV; magnesium sulfate 4 g in 250 mL D5W loading dose to infuse over 30 min; magnesium sulfate 40 g in 1000 mL LR to infuse at 1 g/hr; nifedipine (Procardia) 10 mg sublingual

1. $\dfrac{25\theta \text{ mg}}{} \left| \dfrac{\text{tablet}}{50\theta \text{ mg}} \right| \dfrac{25}{50} = 0.5 \text{ tablets}$

2. $\dfrac{5 \text{ mg}}{} \left| \dfrac{\text{mL}}{20 \text{ mg}} \right| \dfrac{5}{20} = 0.25 \text{ mL}$

3. $\dfrac{250 \text{ mL}}{30 \text{ min}} \left| \dfrac{6\theta \text{ min}}{1 \text{ hr}} \right| \dfrac{250 \times 6}{3 \times 1} \left| \dfrac{1500}{3} \right. = 500 \dfrac{\text{mL}}{\text{hr}}$

4. $\dfrac{1 \text{ g}}{\text{hr}} \left| \dfrac{100\theta \text{ mL}}{4\theta \text{ g}} \right| \dfrac{1 \times 100}{4} \left| \dfrac{100}{4} \right. = 25 \dfrac{\text{mL}}{\text{hr}}$

5. $\dfrac{10 \text{ mg}}{} \left| \dfrac{\text{capsule}}{10 \text{ mg}} \right| \dfrac{10}{10} = 1 \text{ capsule}$

Case Study 13: **Premature Labor**

Orders requiring calculations: Magnesium sulfate at 2 g/hr; terbutaline (Brethine) 0.25 mg SQ; nifedipine (Procardia) 20 mg; betamethasone 12 mg IM; LR 1000 cc over 8 hr

1. $\dfrac{250 \text{ cc}}{2\theta \text{ min}} \left| \dfrac{6\theta \text{ min}}{1 \text{ hr}} \right| \dfrac{250 \times 6}{2 \times 1} \left| \dfrac{1500}{2} \right. = 750 \dfrac{\text{cc}}{\text{hr}}$

$\dfrac{2 \text{ g}}{\text{hr}} \left| \dfrac{250 \text{ cc}}{4 \text{ g}} \right| \dfrac{2 \times 250}{4} \left| \dfrac{500}{4} \right. = 125 \dfrac{\text{cc}}{\text{hr}}$

2. $\dfrac{0.25 \text{ mg}}{} \left| \dfrac{\text{mL}}{1 \text{ mg}} \right| \dfrac{0.25}{1} = 0.25 \text{ mL}$

3. $\dfrac{2\theta \text{ mg}}{} \left| \dfrac{\text{capsule}}{1\theta \text{ mg}} \right| \dfrac{2}{1} = 2 \text{ capsules}$

4. $\dfrac{12\ \text{mg}}{}\ \bigg|\ \dfrac{\text{mL}}{6\ \text{mg}}\ \bigg|\ \dfrac{12}{6} = 2\ \text{mL}$

5. $\dfrac{1000\ \text{cc}}{8\ \text{hr}}\ \bigg|\ \dfrac{1000}{8} = \dfrac{125\ \text{cc}}{\text{hr}}$

Case Study 14: Cystic Fibrosis

Orders requiring calculations: IV 0.9% normal saline at 75 cc/hr; Tagamet 30 mg PO; clindamycin 10 mg/kg IV; terbutaline 2.5 mg PO; tobramycin 1.5 mg/kg IV

1. $\dfrac{75\ \text{cc}}{\text{hr}}\ \bigg|\ \dfrac{15\ \text{gtt}}{\text{mL}}\ \bigg|\ \dfrac{1\ \text{hr}}{60\ \text{min}}\ \bigg|\ \dfrac{75 \times 15 \times 1}{60}\ \bigg|\ \dfrac{1125}{60} = \dfrac{18.75\ \text{or}\ 19\ \text{gtt}}{\text{min}}$

2. $\dfrac{30\ \text{mg}}{\text{kg/day}}\ \bigg|\ \dfrac{\text{tablet}}{200\ \text{mg}}\ \bigg|\ \dfrac{1\ \text{kg}}{2.2\ \text{lb}}\ \bigg|\ \dfrac{65\ \text{lb}}{}\ \bigg|\ \dfrac{\text{day}}{4\ \text{doses}}\ \bigg|\ \dfrac{3 \times 1 \times 65}{20 \times 2.2 \times 4}\ \bigg|\ \dfrac{195}{176} = \dfrac{1.1\ \text{or}\ 1\ \text{tablet}}{\text{dose}}$

3. $\dfrac{10\ \text{mg}}{\text{kg}}\ \bigg|\ \dfrac{1\ \text{kg}}{2.2\ \text{lb}}\ \bigg|\ \dfrac{65\ \text{lb}}{}\ \bigg|\ \dfrac{10 \times 1 \times 65}{2.2}\ \bigg|\ \dfrac{650}{2.2} = 295.45\ \text{or}\ 295\ \text{mg}$

   $\dfrac{295\ \text{mg}}{}\ \bigg|\ \dfrac{\text{mL}}{150\ \text{mg}}\ \bigg|\ \dfrac{295}{150} = 1.96\ \text{or}\ 2\ \text{mL}$

   $\dfrac{52\ \text{mL}}{20\ \text{min}}\ \bigg|\ \dfrac{60\ \text{min}}{1\ \text{hr}}\ \bigg|\ \dfrac{52 \times 6}{2 \times 1}\ \bigg|\ \dfrac{312}{2} = \dfrac{156\ \text{mL}}{\text{hr}}$

4. $\dfrac{2.5\ \text{mg}}{}\ \bigg|\ \dfrac{\text{tablet}}{2.5\ \text{mg}}\ \bigg|\ \dfrac{2.5}{2.5} = 1\ \text{tablet}$

5. $\dfrac{1.5\ \text{mg}}{\text{kg}}\ \bigg|\ \dfrac{1\ \text{kg}}{2.2\ \text{lb}}\ \bigg|\ \dfrac{65\ \text{lb}}{}\ \bigg|\ \dfrac{1.5 \times 1 \times 65}{2.2}\ \bigg|\ \dfrac{97.5}{2.2} = 44.31\ \text{or}\ 44\ \text{mg}$

   $\dfrac{44\ \text{mg}}{}\ \bigg|\ \dfrac{\text{mL}}{40\ \text{mg}}\ \bigg|\ \dfrac{44}{40} = 1.1\ \text{or}\ 1\ \text{mL}$

   $\dfrac{51\ \text{mL}}{30\ \text{min}}\ \bigg|\ \dfrac{60\ \text{min}}{1\ \text{hr}}\ \bigg|\ \dfrac{51 \times 6}{3 \times 1}\ \bigg|\ \dfrac{306}{3} = \dfrac{102\ \text{mL}}{\text{hr}}$

Case Study 15: Respiratory Syncytial Virus (RSV)

Orders requiring calculations: Acetaminophen elixir 120 mg PO; aminophylline 5 mg/kg to infuse over 30 min and 0.8 mg/kg/hr IV; RespiGam 750 mg/kg IV; Pediapred 1.5 mg/kg/day in three divided doses PO; ampicillin 100 mg/kg/day in divided doses q6h IV

1. $\dfrac{120\ \text{mg}}{}\ \bigg|\ \dfrac{5\ \text{mL}}{120\ \text{mg}}\ \bigg|\ \dfrac{5}{} = 5\ \text{mL}$

2. $\dfrac{5\ \text{mg}}{\text{kg}}\ \bigg|\ \dfrac{1\ \text{kg}}{2.2\ \text{lb}}\ \bigg|\ \dfrac{30\ \text{lb}}{}\ \bigg|\ \dfrac{5 \times 1 \times 30}{2.2}\ \bigg|\ \dfrac{150}{2.2} = 68.18\ \text{or}\ 68.2\ \text{mg}$

   $\dfrac{68.2\ \text{mg}}{30\ \text{min}}\ \bigg|\ \dfrac{100\ \text{mL}}{250\ \text{mg}}\ \bigg|\ \dfrac{60\ \text{min}}{1\ \text{hr}}\ \bigg|\ \dfrac{68.2 \times 10 \times 6}{3 \times 25 \times 1}\ \bigg|\ \dfrac{4092}{75} = \dfrac{54.56\ \text{or}\ 54.6\ \text{mL}}{\text{hr}}$

   $\dfrac{0.8\ \text{mg}}{\text{kg/hr}}\ \bigg|\ \dfrac{100\ \text{mL}}{250\ \text{mg}}\ \bigg|\ \dfrac{1\ \text{kg}}{2.2\ \text{lb}}\ \bigg|\ \dfrac{30\ \text{lb}}{}\ \bigg|\ \dfrac{0.8 \times 100 \times 1 \times 3}{25 \times 2.2}\ \bigg|\ \dfrac{240}{55} = \dfrac{4.36\ \text{or}\ 4.4\ \text{mL}}{\text{hr}}$

3. $\dfrac{750\ \text{mg}}{\text{kg}}\ \bigg|\ \dfrac{1\ \text{kg}}{2.2\ \text{lb}}\ \bigg|\ \dfrac{30\ \text{lb}}{}\ \bigg|\ \dfrac{750 \times 1 \times 30}{2.2}\ \bigg|\ \dfrac{22,500}{2.2} = 10,227.27\ \text{or}\ 10,227.3\ \text{mg}$

4. $\dfrac{1.5\ \text{mg}}{\text{kg/day}}\ \bigg|\ \dfrac{5\ \text{mL}}{15\ \text{mg}}\ \bigg|\ \dfrac{1\ \text{kg}}{2.2\ \text{lb}}\ \bigg|\ \dfrac{30\ \text{lb}}{}\ \bigg|\ \dfrac{\text{day}}{3\ \text{doses}}\ \bigg|\ \dfrac{1.5 \times 5 \times 1 \times 30}{15 \times 2.2 \times 3}\ \bigg|\ \dfrac{225}{99} = \dfrac{2.27\ \text{or}\ 2.3\ \text{mL}}{\text{dose}}$

5. $\dfrac{100\ \text{mg}}{\text{kg/day}}\ \bigg|\ \dfrac{1\ \text{kg}}{2.2\ \text{lb}}\ \bigg|\ \dfrac{30\ \text{lb}}{}\ \bigg|\ \dfrac{\text{day}}{4\ \text{doses}}\ \bigg|\ \dfrac{100 \times 1 \times 30}{2.2 \times 4}\ \bigg|\ \dfrac{3000}{8.8} = \dfrac{340.9\ \text{or}\ 341\ \text{mg}}{\text{dose}}$

   $\dfrac{341\ \text{mg}}{}\ \bigg|\ \dfrac{10\ \text{mL}}{1\ \text{g}}\ \bigg|\ \dfrac{1\ \text{g}}{1000\ \text{mg}}\ \bigg|\ \dfrac{341 \times 1 \times 1}{1 \times 100}\ \bigg|\ \dfrac{341}{100} = 3.41\ \text{or}\ 3.4\ \text{mL}$

   $\dfrac{53\ \text{cc}}{30\ \text{min}}\ \bigg|\ \dfrac{60\ \text{min}}{1\ \text{hr}}\ \bigg|\ \dfrac{53 \times 6}{3 \times 1}\ \bigg|\ \dfrac{318}{3} = \dfrac{106\ \text{cc}}{\text{hr}}$

Case Study 16: **Leukemia**

Orders requiring calculations: IV D5W/NS with 20 mEq KCl 1000 mL over 8 hours; allopurinol 200 mg PO; Fortaz 1 g IV; aztreonam 2 g IV; Flagyl 500 mg IV

1. $\dfrac{1000 \text{ mL}}{8 \text{ hr}} \mid \dfrac{1000}{8} = \dfrac{125 \text{ mL}}{\text{hr}}$

2. $\dfrac{200 \text{ mg}}{} \mid \dfrac{\text{tablet}}{100 \text{ mg}} \mid \dfrac{2}{1} = 2 \text{ tablets}$

3. $\dfrac{1 \text{ g}}{} \mid \dfrac{10 \text{ mL}}{1 \text{ g}} = 10 \text{ mL}$

   $\dfrac{60 \text{ mL}}{30 \text{ min}} \mid \dfrac{60 \text{ min}}{1 \text{ hr}} \mid \dfrac{60 \times 6}{3 \times 1} \mid \dfrac{360}{3} = \dfrac{120 \text{ mL}}{\text{hr}}$

4. $\dfrac{2 \text{ g}}{} \mid \dfrac{10 \text{ mL}}{2 \text{ g}} = 10 \text{ mL}$

   $\dfrac{110 \text{ mL}}{60 \text{ min}} \mid \dfrac{60 \text{ min}}{1 \text{ hr}} \mid \dfrac{110}{1} = \dfrac{110 \text{ mL}}{\text{hr}}$

5. $\dfrac{500 \text{ mg}}{1 \text{ hr}} \mid \dfrac{100 \text{ mL}}{500 \text{ mg}} \mid \dfrac{100}{1} = \dfrac{100 \text{ mL}}{\text{hr}}$

Case Study 17: **Sepsis**

Orders requiring calculations: NG breast milk with sterile water 120 cc per feeding; IV D10 and 20% lipids 120 cc/kg/day; aminophylline 5 mg/kg IV q6h; cefotaxime 50 mg/kg q12h; vancomycin 10 mg/kg/dose q12h

1. $\dfrac{120 \text{ cc}}{\text{day}} \mid \dfrac{\text{day}}{24 \text{ hr}} \mid \dfrac{3 \text{ hr}}{\text{feeding}} \mid \dfrac{120 \times 3}{24} \mid \dfrac{360}{24} = \dfrac{15 \text{ cc}}{\text{feeding}}$

2. $\dfrac{120 \text{ mL}}{\text{kg/day}} \mid \dfrac{\text{day}}{24 \text{ hr}} \mid \dfrac{1 \text{ kg}}{1000 \text{ g}} \mid 2005 \text{ g} \mid \dfrac{12 \times 1 \times 2005}{24 \times 100} \mid \dfrac{24{,}060}{2400} = \dfrac{10.025 \text{ or } 10 \text{ mL}}{\text{hr}}$

3. $\dfrac{5 \text{ mg}}{\text{kg}} \mid \dfrac{1 \text{ kg}}{1000 \text{ g}} \mid 2005 \text{ g} \mid \dfrac{5 \times 1 \times 2005}{1000} \mid \dfrac{10025}{1000} = 10.025 \text{ or } 10 \text{ mg}$

   $\dfrac{10 \text{ mg}}{5 \text{ min}} \mid \dfrac{10 \text{ mL}}{50 \text{ mg}} \mid \dfrac{60 \text{ min}}{1 \text{ hr}} \mid \dfrac{10 \times 10 \times 6}{5 \times 5 \times 1} \mid \dfrac{600}{25} = \dfrac{24 \text{ mL}}{\text{hr}}$

4. $\dfrac{50 \text{ mg}}{\text{kg}} \mid \dfrac{1 \text{ kg}}{1000 \text{ g}} \mid 2005 \text{ g} \mid \dfrac{5 \times 1 \times 2005}{100} \mid \dfrac{10025}{100} = 100.25 \text{ or } 100 \text{ mg}$

   $\dfrac{100 \text{ mg}}{30 \text{ min}} \mid \dfrac{\text{mL}}{40 \text{ mg}} \mid \dfrac{60 \text{ min}}{1 \text{ hr}} \mid \dfrac{10 \times 6}{3 \times 4 \times 1} \mid \dfrac{60}{12} = \dfrac{5 \text{ mL}}{\text{hr}}$

5. $\dfrac{10 \text{ mg}}{\text{kg/dose}} \mid \dfrac{1 \text{ kg}}{1000 \text{ g}} \mid 2005 \text{ g} \mid \dfrac{1 \times 1 \times 2005}{100} \mid \dfrac{2005}{100} = \dfrac{20.05 \text{ or } 20 \text{ mg}}{\text{dose}}$

   $\dfrac{20 \text{ mg}}{1 \text{ hr}} \mid \dfrac{1 \text{ mL}}{5 \text{ mg}} \mid \dfrac{20 \times 1}{1 \times 5} \mid \dfrac{20}{5} = \dfrac{4 \text{ mL}}{\text{hr}}$

Case Study 18: **Bronchopulmonary Dysplasia**

Orders requiring calculations: NG feedings with Special Care with Iron 120 KCal/kg/day; chlorothiazide 10 mg/kg/day; Fer-In-Sol 2 mg/kg/day; vitamin E 25 units/kg/day in divided doses q12h; caffeine citrate 5 mg/kg/dose daily

1. $\dfrac{120 \text{ kcal}}{\text{kg/day}} \mid \dfrac{1 \text{ kg}}{1000 \text{ g}} \mid 996 \text{ g} \mid \dfrac{12 \times 1 \times 996}{100} \mid \dfrac{11{,}952}{100} = \dfrac{119.52 \text{ or } 120 \text{ kcal}}{\text{day}}$

   $\dfrac{120 \text{ kcal}}{\text{day}} \mid \dfrac{\text{oz}}{24 \text{ kcal}} \mid \dfrac{30 \text{ cc}}{1 \text{ oz}} \mid \dfrac{120 \times 30}{24 \times 1} \mid \dfrac{3600}{24} = \dfrac{150 \text{ cc}}{\text{day}}$

2. $\dfrac{10 \text{ mg}}{\text{kg/day}} \mid \dfrac{1 \text{ kg}}{1000 \text{ g}} \mid 996 \text{ g} \mid \dfrac{1 \times 1 \times 996}{100} \mid \dfrac{996}{100} = \dfrac{9.96 \text{ or } 10 \text{ mg}}{\text{day}}$

   $\dfrac{10 \text{ mg}}{\text{day}} \mid \dfrac{5 \text{ mL}}{250 \text{ mg}} \mid \dfrac{1 \times 5}{25} \mid \dfrac{5}{25} = \dfrac{0.2 \text{ mL}}{\text{day}}$

3. $\dfrac{2 \text{ mg}}{\text{kg/day}} \mid \dfrac{1 \text{ kg}}{1000 \text{ g}} \mid 996 \text{ g} \mid \dfrac{2 \times 1 \times 996}{1000} \mid \dfrac{1992}{1000} = \dfrac{1.99 \text{ or } 2 \text{ mg}}{\text{day}}$

   $\dfrac{2 \text{ mg}}{\text{day}} \mid \dfrac{0.6 \text{ mL}}{15 \text{ mg}} \mid \dfrac{2 \times 0.6}{15} \mid \dfrac{1.2}{15} = \dfrac{0.08 \text{ mL}}{\text{day}}$

4. $\dfrac{25\,\text{units}}{\text{kg/day}}\left|\dfrac{1\,\text{kg}}{1000\,\text{g}}\right|\dfrac{996\,\text{g}}{}\left|\dfrac{\text{day}}{2\,\text{doses}}\right|\dfrac{25\times1\times996}{1000\times2}\left|\dfrac{24{,}900}{2000}\right.=\dfrac{12.45\ \text{or}\ 12.5\ \text{units}}{\text{dose}}$

$\dfrac{12.5\,\text{units}}{\text{dose}}\left|\dfrac{\text{mL}}{67\,\text{units}}\right|\dfrac{12.5}{67}=\dfrac{0.18\ \text{or}\ 0.2\ \text{mL}}{\text{dose}}$

5. $\dfrac{5\,\text{mg}}{\text{kg/day}}\left|\dfrac{1\,\text{kg}}{1000\,\text{g}}\right|\dfrac{996\,\text{g}}{}\left|\dfrac{\text{day}}{4\,\text{doses}}\right|\dfrac{5\times1\times996}{1000\times4}\left|\dfrac{4980}{4000}\right.=\dfrac{1.24\ \text{or}\ 1.2\ \text{mg}}{\text{dose}}$

$\dfrac{1.2\,\text{mg}}{\text{dose}}\left|\dfrac{\text{mL}}{10\,\text{mg}}\right|\dfrac{1.2}{10}=\dfrac{0.12\ \text{or}\ 0.1\ \text{mL}}{\text{dose}}$

Case Study 19: **Cerebral Palsy**

Orders requiring calculations: Lactulose 3 g PO tid; Depakote 30 mg/kg/day PO in three divided doses; diazapam 2.5 mg PO daily; chlorothiazide 250 mg PO daily; Dilantin 5 mg/kg/day PO in three divided doses

1. $\dfrac{3\,\text{g}}{}\left|\dfrac{15\,\text{mL}}{10\,\text{g}}\right|\dfrac{3\times15}{10}\left|\dfrac{45}{10}\right.=4.5\ \text{or}\ 5\ \text{mL}$

2. $\dfrac{30\,\text{mg}}{\text{kg/day}}\left|\dfrac{38\,\text{kg}}{3\,\text{doses}}\right|\dfrac{\text{day}}{}\left|\dfrac{30\times38}{3}\right|\dfrac{1140}{3}=\dfrac{380\ \text{mg}}{\text{dose}}$

$\dfrac{380\,\text{mg}}{}\left|\dfrac{\text{tablet}}{125\,\text{mg}}\right|\dfrac{380}{125}=3.04\ \text{or}\ 3\ \text{tablets}$

3. $\dfrac{2.5\,\text{mg}}{}\left|\dfrac{\text{tablet}}{5\,\text{mg}}\right|\dfrac{2.5}{5}=0.5\ \text{tablet}$

4. $\dfrac{250\,\text{mg}}{}\left|\dfrac{\text{tablet}}{250\,\text{mg}}\right|\dfrac{250}{250}=1\ \text{tablet}$

5. $\dfrac{5\,\text{mg}}{\text{kg/day}}\left|\dfrac{38\,\text{kg}}{3\,\text{dose}}\right|\dfrac{\text{day}}{}\left|\dfrac{5\,\text{mL}}{125\,\text{mg}}\right|\dfrac{5\times38\times5}{3\times125}\left|\dfrac{950}{375}\right.=\dfrac{2.53\ \text{or}\ 2.5\ \text{mL}}{\text{dose}}$

Case Study 20: **Hyperbilirubinemia**

Orders requiring calculations: Albumin 5% infusion 1 g/kg 1 hr before exchange; ampicillin 100 mg/kg/dose IV q12h; gentamicin 2.5 mg/kg/dose IV q12h; 120 cc/kg/day formula; IV D10W 120 cc/kg/day

1. $\dfrac{1\,\text{g}}{\text{kg}}\left|\dfrac{1\,\text{kg}}{1000\,\text{g}}\right|\dfrac{2210\,\text{g}}{}\left|\dfrac{1\times1\times221}{100}\right|\dfrac{221}{100}=2.21\ \text{or}\ 2.2\ \text{g}$

2. $\dfrac{100\,\text{mg}}{\text{kg/dose}}\left|\dfrac{1\,\text{kg}}{1000\,\text{g}}\right|\dfrac{2210\,\text{g}}{}\left|\dfrac{1\times221}{1}\right|\dfrac{221}{1}=\dfrac{221\ \text{mg}}{\text{dose}}$

$\dfrac{221\,\text{mg}}{}\left|\dfrac{5\,\text{mL}}{250\,\text{mg}}\right|\dfrac{221\times5}{250}\left|\dfrac{1105}{250}\right.=4.42\ \text{or}\ 4.4\ \text{mL}$

3. $\dfrac{4\,\text{mg}}{\text{kg/dose}}\left|\dfrac{1\,\text{kg}}{1000\,\text{g}}\right|\dfrac{2210\,\text{g}}{}\left|\dfrac{4\times1\times221}{100}\right|\dfrac{884}{100}=\dfrac{8.84\ \text{or}\ 8.8\ \text{mg}}{\text{dose}}$

$\dfrac{8.8\,\text{mg}}{}\left|\dfrac{\text{mL}}{2\,\text{mg}}\right|\dfrac{8.8}{2}=4.4\ \text{mL}$

4. $\dfrac{120\,\text{cc}}{\text{kg/day}}\left|\dfrac{1\,\text{kg}}{1000\,\text{g}}\right|\dfrac{2210\,\text{g}}{}\left|\dfrac{12\times1\times221}{10}\right|\dfrac{2652}{10}=\dfrac{265.2\ \text{or}\ 265\ \text{cc}}{\text{day}}$

5. $\dfrac{120\,\text{cc}}{\text{kg/day}}\left|\dfrac{1\,\text{kg}}{1000\,\text{g}}\right|\dfrac{\text{day}}{24\,\text{hr}}\left|\dfrac{12\times1\times221}{10\times24}\right|\dfrac{2652}{240}=\dfrac{11.05\ \text{or}\ 11\ \text{cc}}{\text{hr}}$

Case Study 21: **Spontaneous Abortion**

Orders requiring calculations: Rhogam 300 mcg IM; IV D5/0.9% NS at 100 cc/hr; oxytocin (Pitocin) 10 units infused at 20 mL/min; meperidine 50 mg IM q4h; ibuprofen 400 mg PO

1. $\dfrac{300\text{ mcg} \mid 1\text{ ml} \mid 1}{\mid 300\text{ mcg} \mid} = 1\text{ mL}$

2. $\dfrac{100\text{ mL} \mid 15\text{ gtt} \mid 1\text{ hr} \mid 10\times15\times1 \mid 150}{\text{hr} \mid \text{mL} \mid 60\text{ min} \mid 6 \mid 6} = \dfrac{25\text{ gtt}}{\text{min}}$

3. $\dfrac{20\text{ mU} \mid 500\text{ mL} \mid 1\text{ U} \mid 60\text{ min} \mid 2\times5\times1\times6 \mid 60}{\text{min} \mid 10\text{ U} \mid 1000\text{ mU} \mid 1\text{ hr} \mid 1\times1\times1 \mid 1} = \dfrac{60\text{ mL}}{\text{hr}}$

4. $\dfrac{50\text{ mg} \mid \text{mL} \mid 5}{\mid 100\text{ mg} \mid 10} = 0.5\text{ mL}$

5. $\dfrac{400\text{ mg} \mid \text{tablet} \mid 4}{\mid 200\text{ mg} \mid 2} = 2\text{ tablets}$

Case Study 22: **Bipolar Disorder**

IV 0.9% NS at 75 cc/hr; lithium 300 mg, lithium 300 mg; clonazepam 0.5 mg; clonazepam 1 mg; doxepin 25 mg

1. $\dfrac{75\text{ mL} \mid 20\text{ gtt} \mid 1\text{ hr} \mid 75\times2\times1 \mid 150}{\text{hr} \mid \text{mL} \mid 60\text{ min} \mid 6 \mid 6} = \dfrac{25\text{ gtt}}{\text{min}}$

2. $\dfrac{300\text{ mg} \mid \text{capsule} \mid 30}{\mid 150\text{ mg} \mid 15} = 2\text{ capsules}$

3. $\dfrac{0.5\text{ mg} \mid \text{tablet} \mid 0.5}{\mid 0.5\text{ mg} \mid 0.5} = 1\text{ tablet}$

4. $\dfrac{1\text{ mg} \mid \text{tablet} \mid 1}{\mid 0.5\text{ mg} \mid 0.5} = 2\text{ tablets}$

5. $\dfrac{50\text{ mg} \mid \text{tablet} \mid 50}{\mid 25\text{ mg} \mid 25} = 2\text{ tablets}$

Case Study 23: **Anorexia Nervosa**

IV 1000 cc/8 hr; olanzapine (Zyprexa) 10 mg; fluoxetine (Prozac) 60 mg/day; Amitriptyline 25 mg; Cyproheptadine 32 mg/day

1. $\dfrac{1000\text{ cc}}{8\text{ hr}} = \dfrac{125\text{ cc}}{\text{hr}}$

2. $\dfrac{10\text{ mg} \mid \text{tablets} \mid 10}{\mid 5\text{ mg} \mid 5} = 2\text{ tablets}$

3. $\dfrac{60\text{ mg} \mid 5\text{ mL} \mid 6\times5 \mid 30}{\mid 20\text{ mg} \mid 2 \mid 2} = 15\text{ mL}$

4. $\dfrac{25\text{ mg} \mid 5\text{ mL} \mid 25\times5 \mid 125}{\mid 10\text{ mg} \mid 10 \mid 10} = 12.5\text{ mL}$

5. $\dfrac{32\text{ mg} \mid \text{day}}{\text{day} \mid 4\text{ doses}} = \dfrac{8\text{ mg}}{\text{dose}}$

$\dfrac{8\text{ mg} \mid 5\text{ mL} \mid 8\times5 \mid 40}{\mid 2\text{ mg} \mid 2 \mid 2} = 20\text{ mL}$

Case Study 24: **Clinical Depression**

IV 100 mL/hr; glycopyrrolate (Robinul) 4.4 mcg/kg; Zoloft 50 mg PO qAM; Sinequan 25 mg PO tid; Parnate 30 mg/day PO in 2 divided doses

1. $\dfrac{100\text{ mL} \mid 10\text{ gtt} \mid 1\text{ hr} \mid 10\times10 \mid 100}{\text{hr} \mid \text{mL} \mid 60\text{ min} \mid 6 \mid 6} = \dfrac{16.6\text{ or }17\text{ gtt}}{\text{min}}$

2. $\dfrac{4.4\text{ mcg} \mid \text{mL} \mid 1\text{ kg} \mid 175\text{ lb} \mid 4.4\times1\times175 \mid 770}{\text{kg} \mid 200\text{ mcg} \mid 2.2\text{ lb} \mid \mid 200\times2.2 \mid 440} = 1.75\text{ or }1.8\text{ mL}$

3. $\dfrac{50\text{ mg} \mid \text{tablet} \mid 5}{\mid 50\text{ mg} \mid 5} = 1\text{ tablet}$

4. $\dfrac{25 \ \cancel{mg} \ | \ \boxed{capsule} \ | \ 25}{\ | \ 25 \ \cancel{mg} \ | \ 25} = 1 \text{ capsule}$

5. $\dfrac{30 \ \boxed{mg} \ | \ \cancel{day} \ | \ 30}{\cancel{day} \ | \ 2 \ \boxed{doses} \ | \ 2} = \dfrac{15 \text{ mg}}{\text{dose}}$

$\dfrac{15 \ \cancel{mg} \ | \ \boxed{tablet} \ | \ 15}{\ | \ 10 \ \cancel{mg} \ | \ 10} = 1.5 \text{ tablets}$

Case Study 25: Alzheimer's Disease

IV 1000 mL/8 hr; donepezil (Aricept) 5 mg; thioridazine (Mellaril) 25 mg; imipramine (Tofranil) 50 mg; temazepam (Restoril) 7.5 mg

1. $\dfrac{1000 \ \cancel{mL} \ | \ 10 \ \boxed{gtt} \ | \ 1 \ \cancel{hr} \ | \ 100 \times 10 \times 1 \ | \ 1000}{8 \ \cancel{hr} \ | \ \cancel{mL} \ | \ 60 \ \boxed{min} \ | \ 8 \times 6 \ | \ 48} = \dfrac{20.83 \text{ or } 21}{\text{min}} \ \text{gtt}$

2. $\dfrac{5 \ \cancel{mg} \ | \ \boxed{tablet} \ | \ 5}{\ | \ 5 \ \cancel{mg} \ | \ 5} = 1 \text{ tablet}$

3. $\dfrac{25 \ \cancel{mg} \ | \ \boxed{tablet} \ | \ 25}{\ | \ 25 \ \cancel{mg} \ | \ 25} = 1 \text{ tablet}$

4. $\dfrac{50 \ \cancel{mg} \ | \ \boxed{tablet} \ | \ 50}{\ | \ 25 \ \cancel{mg} \ | \ 25} = 2 \text{ tablets}$

5. $\dfrac{7.5 \ \cancel{mg} \ | \ \boxed{tablet} \ | \ 7.5}{\ | \ 15 \ \cancel{mg} \ | \ 15} = 0.5 \text{ tablet}$

Comprehensive Post-Test

Comprehensive Post-Test

Name _____ **Date** _____

1. Order: Phenobarbital 60 mg PO daily for seizures

   Supply on hand: Phenobarbital 30 mg/tablet

   ▶ **How many tablets will you give?** _____

2. Order: Chloral hydrate 250 mg PO 30 minutes before hs as sedative

   Supply on hand: Chloral hydrate 250 mg/5 mL

   ▶ **How many milliliters will you give?** _____

3. Order: Digitoxin 0.3 mg PO daily for maintenance dose after digitalization

   Supply on hand: Digitoxin 100-mcg tablets

   ▶ **How many tablets will you give?** _____

4. Order: Potassium chloride 20 mEq PO tid for hypokalemia

   Supply: Potassium chloride 40 mEq/15 mL

   ▶ **How many teaspoons will you give?** _____

5. Order: 500 mL D5W to infuse over 12 hours

   Drop factor: 60 gtt/mL

   ▶ **Calculate the number of drops per minute.** _____

6. Order: Heparin 1500 units/hr for thrombophlebitis

   Supply: Heparin 25,000 units/500 cc

   ▶ **Calculate cc/hr to set the IV pump.** _____

7. Order: Infuse heparin at 20 cc/hr for thrombophlebitis

   Supply: Heparin 25,000 units in 250 cc

   ▶ **How many units/hr is the patient receiving?** _____

8. Order: Infuse bolus of 0.9% NS at 100 gtt/min

   Supply: 250 mL 0.9% NS with 60 gtt/mL tubing

   ▶ **How many hours will it take to infuse the IV bolus?** _____

9. Order: Fluconazole 200 mg IVPB over 60 minutes for systemic candidal infections

   Supply: Fluconazole 200 mg/100 mL with 20 gtt/mL tubing

   ▶ **Calculate the number of drops per minute.** _____

10. Order: Furosemide 2 mg/kg PO daily for congestive heart failure

    Supply: Furosemide 10 mg/mL oral solution

    ▶ **How many milliliters will you give a child weighing 10 lb?** _____

11. Order: Neupogen 6 mcg/kg SQ twice daily for chronic neutropenia

    Supply: Neupogen 300 mcg/mL

    ▶ **How many milliliters will you give a patient weighing 175 lb?** _____

12. Order: Ampicillin 500 mg IV every 6 hours for urinary tract infection

    Supply: Ampicillin 1-g vial

    Nursing drug reference: Reconstitute each 1-g vial with 10 mL of sterile water and further dilute in 50 mL of 0.9% NS and infuse over 15 minutes.

    ▶ **How many milliliters will you draw from the vial after reconstitution?** _____

    ▶ **Calculate the milliliters per hour to set the IV pump.** _____

    ▶ **Calculate the drops per minute with a drop factor of 10 gtt/mL.** _____

13. Order: Acyclovir 10 mg/kg IV every 8 hours for varicella zoster in immunosuppressed patient weighing 140 lb

    Supply: Acyclovir 1-g vial.

    Nursing drug reference: Reconstitute each 1-g vial with 10 mL of sterile water and further dilute in 100 mL of 0.9% NS and infuse over 1 hour.

    ▶ **How many milliliters will you draw from the vial after reconstitution?** _____

▶ **Calculate the milliliters per hour to set the IV pump.** ——————

▶ **Calculate the drops per minute with a drop factor of 10 gtt/mL.** ——————

14. Order: Epinephrine 1 mcg/min IV for bradycardia

    Supply: Epinephrine 1 mg/250 mL 0.9% NS

    ▶ **Calculate the milliliters per hour to set the IV pump.** ——————

15. Order: Isuprel 5 mcg/min IV for heart block

    Supply: Isuprel 2 mg in 500 mL D5W

    ▶ **Calculate the milliliters per hour to set the IV pump.** ——————

16. Order: Dobutamine 2.5 mcg/kg/min IV for management of heart failure for a patient weighing 130 lb

    Supply: Dobutamine 250 mg in 1000 mL of 0.9% NS

    ▶ **Calculate the milliliters per hour to set the IV pump.** ——————

17. Order: Dopamine 10 mcg/kg/min IV for management of hypotension secondary to decreased cardiac output for a patient weighing 120 lb

    Supply: Dopamine 400 mg in 500 mL D5W

    ▶ **Calculate the milliliters per hour to set the IV pump.** ——————

18. Order: Aminophylline is infusing at 24 mL/hr for respiratory distress for a patient weighing 80 kg

    Supply: Aminophylline is 250 mg in 250 mL in D5W

    ▶ **How many mg/kg/hr is the patient receiving?** ——————

19. Order: Amrinone infusing at 47 mL/hr for a patient weighing 100 kg for short-term treatment of congestive heart failure

    Supply: Amrinone 100 mg/100 mL 0.45% NS

    ▶ **How many mcg/kg/min is the patient receiving?** ——————

20. Order: Aminophylline loading dose of 5.6 mg/kg to infuse over 30 minutes for a patient weighing 50 kg followed by 0.6 mg/kg/hr maintenance dose for COPD

Supply: Aminophylline 500 mg in 500 mL of D5W

▶ **How many milliliters per hour will you set the IV pump for the loading dose?** _____

▶ **How many milliliters per hour will you set the IV pump for the maintenance dose?** _____

Educational Theory of Dimensional Analysis

Dimensional analysis is a problem-solving method based on the principles of cognitive theory. Bruner (1960) theorized that learning is dependent on how information is structured, organized, and conceptualized. He proposed a cognitive learning model that emphasized the acquisition, organization (structure), understanding, and transfer of knowledge—focusing on "how" to learn, rather than "what" to learn. Learning involves associations established according to the principles of continuity and repetition.

Dimensional analysis (also called factor-label method, conversion-factor method, units analysis, and quantity calculus) provides a systematic way to set up problems and helps to organize and evaluate data. Hein (1983) emphasized that dimensional analysis gives a clear understanding of the principles of the problem-solving method that correlates with the ability to verbalize what steps are taken leading to critical thinking. He described dimensional analysis as a useful method for solving a variety of chemistry, physics, mathematics, and daily life problems. He identified that dimensional analysis is often the problem-solving method of choice because it provides a straightforward way to set up problems, gives a clear understanding of the principles of the problem, helps the learner to organize and evaluate data, and assists in identifying errors if the setup of the problem is incorrect.

Goodstein (1983) described dimensional analysis as a problem-solving method that is very simple to understand, reduces errors, and requires less conceptual reasoning power to understand than does the ratio–proportion method. She expressed that "even though the ratio–proportion method was at one time the primary problem-solving method, it has been largely replaced by a dimensional analysis approach in most introductory chemistry textbooks . . . this method condenses multi-step problems into one orderly extended solution."

Peters (1986) identified dimensional analysis as a method used for solving not only chemistry problems but also a variety of other mathematical problems that require conversions. He defined dimensional analysis as a method that can be used whenever two quantities are directly proportional to each other and one quantity must be converted to the other using a conversion factor or conversion relationship.

Literature that has examined the quality of higher education and professional education in the United States (National Institute of Education, 1984) recommends that educators increase the emphasis of the intellectual skills of problem solving and critical thinking. Also recommended is an increased emphasis on the mastery of concepts rather than specific facts. Other literature on curriculum revolution in nursing (Bevis, 1988; Lindeman, 1989; Tanner, 1988) recommends that learning not be characterized merely as a change in behavior or the acquisition of facts, but in seeing and *understanding* the significance of the whole. Because it focuses on "how" to learn, rather than "what" to learn, dimensional analysis supports conceptual mastery and higher-level thinking skills that have become the core of the curriculum change that is sweeping through all levels of education and, most importantly, nursing education.

APPENDIX

BIBLIOGRAPHY

Bevis, E. (1988). New directions for a new age. In National League for Nursing, *Curriculum revolution: Mandate for change* (pp. 27–52). New York: National League for Nursing (Pub. No. 15–2224).

Bruner, J. (1960). *The process of education.* New York: Random House.

Craig, G. (1995). The effects of dimensional analysis on the medication dosage calculation abilities of nursing students. *Nurse Educator, 20*(3), 14–18.

Craig, G. P. (1997). The effectiveness of dimensional analysis as a problem-solving method for medication calculations from the nursing student perspective. Unpublished doctoral dissertation, Drake University, Des Moines, IA.

Goodstein, M. (1983). Reflections upon mathematics in the introductory chemistry course. *Journal of Chemical Education, 60*(8), 665–667.

Hein, M. (1983). *Foundations of chemistry* (4th ed.). Encino, CA: Dickenson Publishing Company.

Lindeman, C. (1989). Curriculum revolution: Reconceptualizing clinical nursing education. *Nursing and Health Care, 10*(1), 23–28.

National Institute of Education. (1984). *Involvement in learning: Realizing the potential of American higher education.* Washington, DC: National Institute of Education.

Peters, E. (1986). *Introduction to chemical principles* (4th ed.). Saratoga, CA: Saunders College Publishing.

Tanner, C. (1988). Curriculum revolution: The practice mandate. *Nursing and Health Care, 9*(8), 426–430.

Index

Page numbers followed by *f* refer to figures; page numbers followed by *t* refer to tables.

A

Abortion, spontaneous, case study of, 231
Acetaminophen. *See* Tylenol (acetaminophen)
Acquired immunodeficiency syndrome (AIDS), case study of, 216
Achromycin (tetracycline), dosage calculation for, 68
Acyclovir, dosage calculation for, 248–249
   involving drop factor, 125
   involving reconstitution, 120
Adalat, dosage calculation for, one-factor, 167, 167*f*
Administration routes, for medications, 74–86
   enteral, 74–80
   intravenous, 112–116
     drop factors in, 116–120
     intermittent, 120–123
   parenteral, 80–86
Advil (ibuprofen), dosage calculation for, 64–65
AIDS (acquired immunodeficiency syndrome), case study of, 216
Alprazolam. *See* Xanax (alprazolam)
Alzheimer's disease, case study of, 234
Aminophylline
   administration of, intravenous, 114–116
   dosage calculation for, 195, 249, 250
     three-factor, 151, 156
Ampicillin. *See* Unasyn (ampicillin)
Amrinone, dosage calculation for, 249
   three-factor, 150, 156, 156*f*
Ancef (cefazolin), dosage calculation for
   in children, 130, 130*f*
   involving reconstitution, 111, 111*f*
   three-factor, 145, 145*f*, 195, 195*f*
Anemia sickle-cell, case study of, 217
Anorexia nervosa, case study of, 232–233
Apothecary measurement system, 31, 32*f*
   abbreviations for, 31–32, 32*f*
   metric equivalents for, 34*t*
Arabic numbers, 4–7, 16
Arithmetic, for calculation of drug dosage, review of, 3–18
Ascorbic acid, dosage calculation for, 193
Aspirin, dosage calculation for, 63–64
   administration of, 61
Atropine sulfate
   administration of, parenteral, 85, 85*f*
   dosage calculation for, 193
     involving weight, 106, 106*f*
     two-factor, 179, 179*f*

Augmentin, dosage calculation for, 89, 89*f*
   in children, 129, 129*f*
   one-factor, 171, 171*f*
Azactam, administration of, intravenous, 130, 130*f*
Azulfidine, dosage calculation for, one-factor, 176, 176*f*

B

Benadryl (diphenhydramine), dosage calculation for, three-factor, 191
Bipolar disorder, case study of, 232
Body weight
   medication problems involving, 104–108
     three-factor, 137–158
   and titration, 138
Bone marrow transplantation, case study of, 218–219
Bretylium, dosage calculation for, three-factor, 149, 149*f*
Bronchopulmonary dysplasia, case study of, 228–229

C

Caplets, administration of, 66–67, 74
Capsules, administration of, 68, 75
Carbamazepine. *See* Tegretol (carbamazepine)
Cefazolin. *See* Ancef (cefazolin)
Cefotaxime. *See* Claforan (cefotaxime)
Ceptaz, dosage calculation for, two-factor, 190, 190*f*
Cerebral palsy, case study of, 229–230
Children, medication problems involving, body weight and, 106–108, 138–156, 179–180, 190–191, 194–195
Chloral hydrate, dosage calculation for, 247
Chlorpromazine. *See* Thorazine (chlorpromazine)
Chronic obstructive pulmonary disease (COPD), case study of, 214
Cimetidine. *See* Tagamet (cimetidine)
Cipro (ciprofloxacin)
   dosage calculation for, 71, 71*f*
   drug label for, components of, 69*f*
Cirrhosis, case study of, 219
Claforan (cefotaxime), dosage calculation for
   involving reconstitution, 110*f*–111*f*, 110–111
   three-factor, 156, 156*f*
Cleocin, dosage calculation for
   one-factor, 176, 176*f*
   three-factor, 146, 146*f*, 191, 191*f*

Clindamycin
  administration of, by intermittent infusion, 122
  dosage calculation for, three-factor, 156, 156*f*
Clinical depression, case study of, 233–234
Cognitive learning model, and dimensional analysis, 253
Colestid, dosage calculation for, two-factor, 184, 184*f*
Compazine (prochlorperazine)
  administration of, as liquid, 77, 77*f*, 173, 173*f*
  dosage calculation for, one-factor, 82, 82*f*, 168, 168*f*, 173, 173*f*
Congestive heart failure, case study of, 213
Conversion-factor method. *See* Dimensional analysis
Conversion factors
  definition of, 42
  in dimensional analysis, 42–49
  solving problems using, one-factor, 62
COPD (chronic obstructive pulmonary disease), case study of, 214
Cortef, dosage calculation for, two-factor, 184, 184*f*
Cystic fibrosis, case study of, 224–225

D

D5W solution
  administration of, intravenous, drop factor in, 118–120, 124–125, 182, 196
  dosage calculation for, 247
  intermittent infusion of, 129
Decimals, 11–14
  conversion of fractions to, 14–15, 18
  division of, 13–14, 17, 20
  multiplication of, 12–13, 17, 20
  rounding of, 11–12, 18, 65
Deep vein thrombosis, case study of, 217–218
Demerol, dosage calculation for, 196
Denominator
  in dimensional analysis, 42, 138
  in fractions, 7
Depo-Provera, dosage calculation for, one-factor, 178, 178*f*
Digits, 4
Digoxin, dosage calculation for, 195, 247
  three-factor, 155, 155*f*
  two-factor, 179, 179*f*
Dilantin, dosage calculation for
  involving reconstitution, 120
  three-factor, 145
Dilaudid
  administration of, as liquid, 79, 79*f*
  dosage calculation for, 195
    two-factor, 179, 179*f*
Diluent, 108
Dimensional analysis
  advantages of, 40
  applications of, 251
  conversion factors in, 42–49

definition of, 42
  denominator in, 42
  in dosage calculation, weight and, 106–108, 138–157
  flexibility of, 143
  numerator in, 42
  in one-factor medication problems, 58–95
  random method of, 67
  sequential method of, 62
  solving problems with, 43–50
  steps in, 42–43
  terms used in, 42
  theory of, 251
Diphenhydramine. *See* Benadryl (diphenhydramine)
Diuril, dosage calculation for, 68
Dividing line, in fractions, 7
Dobutamine, dosage calculation for, 249
  involving body weight, 141–143
Dopamine, dosage calculation for, 198, 249
  three-factor, 147, 147*f*, 148, 150, 192, 192*f*, 193
Dosage
  calculation of, arithmetic needed for, 3–18
  in children. *See* Children
  measurement systems for, 29–36
    apothecary, 31, 31*f*. *See also* Apothecary measurement system
    household, 32–33, 33*f*. *See also* Household measurement system
    metric, 34*t*, 34–35. *See also* Metric system
Drop factors
  definition of, 116
  medication problems involving, 116–120
Drug labels, components of, 68–74
  identification of, 68–70, 69*f*–70*f*
  solving problems with, 71, 71*f*–74*f*

E

Emphysema, case study of, 214
Enteral administration route, 74–80
Epinephrine, dosage calculation for, 247
Epivir, dosage calculation for, two-factor, 187, 188, 188*f*
Epogen, dosage calculation for, 128, 128*f*
  three-factor, 154, 154*f*
Erythromycin
  administration of, by intermittent infusion, 121–122
  dosage calculation for, involving reconstitution, 112, 120
Eskalith (lithium), dosage calculation for, one-factor, 178, 178*f*

F

Factor-label method. *See* Dimensional analysis
Filgrastim (Neupogen), dosage calculation for, three-factor, 154, 154*f*
Five rights of medication administration, 2, 58, 60–62
Fluconazole, dosage calculation for, 248

Fortaz
  administration of, parenteral, 124
  dosage calculation for
    involving reconstitution, 112
    two-factor, 180
Fractions, 7–10
  conversion to decimals, 14–15, 18
  division of, 9–10, 17, 20
  multiplication of, 8–9, 16, 19, 20
Fragmin, dosage calculation for, 175, 175*f*
Furosemide, dosage calculation for, 248
  in children, 127, 127*f*
  involving weight, 106, 106*f*
  one-factor, 173, 173*f*
  three-factor, 144, 144*f*, 151, 191, 191*f*
  two-factor, 127, 127*f*

G

Generic name, 60
Gentamicin, dosage calculation for, 104–105
  three-factor, 156, 191, 194
  two-factor, 180, 183
Given quantity, 42
  solving problems using, 43–49
    one-factor, 62
    three-factor, 138, 140
    two-factor, 104, 140
Glyset, dosage calculation for, one-factor, 177, 177*f*
Gravity flow, in intravenous medication administration, 116

H

Halcion (triazolam)
  dosage calculation for, 72, 72*f*
    one-factor, 165, 165*f*
  drug label for, components of, 79*f*
Hemabate, dosage calculation for, one-factor, 174, 174*f*
Heparin
  administration of
    intravenous, 113, 115, 116, 124, 196
    parenteral, 86, 86*f*
  dosage calculation for, 84, 84*f*, 88, 88*f*, 218, 247
Household measurement system, 32–33, 33*f*
  abbreviations for, 33
  apothecary and metric equivalents for, 34*t*
  conversion to other systems, 33*f*, 33–34
    using dimensional analysis, 42–46
Hydrea, dosage calculation for, three-factor, 192
Hydromorphone
  administration of, parenteral, 85, 85*f*
  dosage calculation for, 94, 94*f*
    one-factor, 172, 172*f*
Hyperbilirubinemia, case study of, 230–231
Hyperemesis gravidarum, case study of, 221–222

I

Ibuprofen (Advil)
  administration of, 61–62
  dosage calculation for, 64–65
Infusion, intermittent, of intravenous medications, 120–123
Inocor, dosage calculation for, three-factor, 148, 193
Insulin
  administration of, 80, 80*f*, 86, 86*f*, 88, 88*f*
    syringes for, 80, 80*f*
  regular, dosage calculation for, 197
Intermittent infusion, of intravenous medications, 120–123
Intravenous medications, administration of, 112–116
  drop factors in, 116–120
  intermittent, 120–123
Isuprel, dosage calculation for, 249
  three-factor, 194

K

KCl. *See* Potassium chloride (KCl)

L

Labels. *See* Drug labels
Labor, premature, case study of, 223–224
Lactulose
  administration of, as liquid, 80, 80*f*
  dosage calculation for, 92, 92*f*
    one-factor, 168, 168*f*
Learning models, cognitive, and dimensional analysis, 253
Lente human insulin, administration of, 83*f*–84*f*, 83–84
Leukemia, case study of, 226–227
  lidocaine, dosage calculation for, two-factor, 180
Lincocin, dosage calculation for, one-factor, 174, 174*f*
Lipids, dosage calculation for, 195
Liquid medication, administration of, 74–80
Lithium. *See* Eskalith (lithium)
Lung cancer, small cell, case study of, 215

M

Macrotubing, 116, 116*t*
Magnesium sulfate, dosage calculation for, 94, 94*f*
  one-factor, 173, 173*f*
Measurement systems, for dosage. *See* Dosage, measurement systems for
Medication
  administration of
    five rights of, 58, 60–62
    routes for. *See* Administration routes
  titration of, body weight and, 136
Medication cups, 75

Medication labels. *See* Drug labels
Medication orders, interpretation of, 58, 60–62
Medication problems
  involving drop factors, 116–120
  one-factor, 62–68
  three-factor, 190–15
    involving weight, 104–130
  two-factor, 99–127, 179–190
    involving reconstitution, 108–112
    involving weight, 104–108
Medications, administration routes for, 70–86
  enteral, 74–80
  intravenous, 112–116
  parenteral, 80–86
Meperidine
  administration of, parenteral, 86, 86*f*
  dosage calculation for, 86, 86*f,* 90, 90*f*
    in children, 128, 128*f*
Methylphenidate. *See* Ritalin (methylphenidate)
Methylprednisolone. *See* Solu-Medrol
    (methylprednisolone)
Metric system, 30*f,* 30–31
  abbreviations for, 31, 31*f*
  apothecary equivalents for, 34*t*
  conversion to other systems, 34–35
    using dimensional analysis, 43–49
Mezlin (mezlocillin)
  dosage calculation for
    involving reconstitution, 107*f*–108*f,* 107–108
    two-factor, 180, 180*f,* 183
  intermittent infusion of, 123
Micronase, dosage calculation for, 91, 91*f*
  one-factor, 177, 177*f*
Microtubing, 116
Mirapex, dosage calculation for, one-factor, 176, 176*f*
Morphine sulfate
  administration of
    intravenous, 82–83, 83*f*
  dosage calculation for
    one-factor, 165, 165*f,* 168, 168*f*
    three-factor, 153, 153*f*
    two-factor, 178
Mycostatin, dosage calculation for, 196

N

Naloxone, dosage calculation for, 95, 95*f*
  one-factor, 169, 169*f*
Neupogen, dosage calculation for, 146
  three-factor, 150
Nipride, dosage calculation for, 193
  three-factor, 148, 149, 151, 192
Nitroglycerin, dosage calculation for, two-factor, 181
Normal saline (NS)
  administration of, intravenous, 114, 181, 196
    drop factor in, 117, 118, 181
  dosage calculation for, 248

NPH human insulin
  administration of, 80, 80*f*
  dosage calculation for, 83, 83*f,* 88, 88*f*
NS. *See* Normal saline (NS)
Numbers, Arabic, 4–7, 16
Numerals, Roman, 4*t,* 4–7, 16
Numerator
  in dimensional analysis, 42, 138
  in fractions, 7

O

One-factor medication problems, 62–67, 165–178
Oral administration, 74–80
Orders, for medication, interpretation of, 60–62
Orinase, dosage calculation for, 87, 87*f*

P

Pain management, case study of, 220
Parenteral administration route, 80–86
Persantine, dosage calculation for, 88, 88*f*
Phenergan, dosage calculation for, involving weight,
    107, 107*f*
Phenobarbital
  administration of, as liquid, 79, 79*f*
  dosage calculation for, 68, 245
Pipracil, dosage calculation for, 198
Pneumonia, case study of, 219–220
Potassium chloride (KCl), dosage calculation for, 197,
    247
  two-factor, 181
Prednisolone, dosage calculation for
  three-factor, 146, 146*f*
Prednisone, dosage calculation for
  one-factor, 166, 166*f,* 171, 171*f*
Preeclampsia, case study of, 222–223
Premature labor, case study of, 223–224
Primaxin, dosage calculation for, involving reconstitu-
    tion, 111
Problem-solving, dimensional analysis in. *See* Dimen-
    sional analysis
Prochlorperazine. *See* Compazine (prochlorperazine)

Q

Quantity
  given, 42
    solving problems using, 42–49
      one-factor, 62
      two-factor, 102
  wanted, 42
    solving problems using, 42–49
      one-factor, 62
Quantity calculus. *See* Dimensional analysis

R

Random method, of dimensional analysis, 62, 67
Reconstitution, medication problems involving, 108–112
Respiratory syncytial virus (RSV) infection, case study of, 225–226
Restoril, dosage calculation for, 68
Rights of medication administration, 2, 58, 60–62
Ritalin (methylphenidate), dosage calculation for, 73, 73f, 90, 90f
Roman numerals, 4t, 4-7, 16
Rounding, of decimals, 11–12, 65
Route of administration. *See* Administration routes

S

Saline, normal
    administration of, intravenous, 114, 118, 181, 196
        drop factor in, 117
    dosage calculation for, 248
Sepsis, case study of, 227–228
Sequential method, of dimensional analysis, 62
Sickle cell anemia, case study of, 217
Small cell lung cancer, case study of, 215–216
Solu-Medrol (methylprednisolone), dosage calculation for, 95, 95f
    involving reconstitution, 109f, 109–110, 110f
    one-factor, 169, 169f
    three-factor, 157
Spontaneous abortion, case study of, 231
Staphcillin, dosage calculation for, 197
Symbols, principles of, 4–5
Syringes, for administration of medication, 80f–81f, 80–81

T

Tablets, administration of, 63–64, 74
Tagamet (cimetidine)
    administration of, as liquid, 76, 76f
    dosage calculation for, 93, 93f
        in children, 138–140, 151
        involving weight, 107f, 107–108, 108f
        one-factor, 76, 76f
        three-factor, 190, 190f
        two-factor, 185, 185f
    drug label for, components of, 69f
Tegretol (carbamazepine)
    administration of, as liquid, 78, 78f
    dosage calculation for, 91, 91f
Temperature
    conversions of, 33, 33f, 34t
    measurements for, 33, 33f
Tetracycline (Achromycin), dosage calculation for, 69

Thorazine (chlorpromazine), dosage calculation for, 68, 87, 87f
    two-factor, 186, 186f
Three-factor medication problems, 137–157, 190–195
Thrombosis, deep vein, case study of, 217–218
Tigan (trimethobenzamide)
    dosage calculation for, 71f, 71–72, 74, 74f, 87, 87f
        one-factor, 165, 165f, 171, 171f
    drug label for, components of, 70, 70f
Time-release capsules, administration of, 75
Titration, body weight and, 136, 138
Tolinase (tolazamide), dosage calculation for, 73, 73f
Trade name, 60
Transplantation, bone barrow, case study of, 218–219
Triazolam. *See* Halcion (triazolam)
Trimethobenzamide. *See* Tigan (trimethobenzamide)
Tuberculin syringe, 81, 81f
Two-factor medication problems, 104–125, 179–180
Tylenol (acetaminophen), dosage calculation for, 66, 92, 92f
    administration of, 61–62
    in children, 124
    one-factor, 166, 166f, 172, 172f

U

Unasyn (ampicillin)
    administration of, by intermittent infusion, 122, 123, 124
    dosage calculation for, 196, 248
        involving reconstitution, 111
        three-factor, 157, 157f
Unit path, 42
    solving problems with, 42–49
        one-factor, 62, 63

V

Vancomycin, dosage calculation for, 196
    in children, 125
    three-factor, 194
    two-factor, 125, 182
Vantin, dosage calculation for, one-factor, 175, 175f
Venoglobulin, dosage calculation for, three-factor, 193
Verapamil, dosage calculation for, in children, 124
Vincristine, dosage calculation for, two-factor, 185, 185f
Vitamin B_{12}, dosage calculation for, 74, 74f
Volume, measurement equivalents for, 32t

W

Wanted quantity, 42, 62
    solving problems using, 43–49
        one-factor, 62
Weight
    medication problems involving, 104–108
        three-factor, 137–157

Weight (*continued*)
 metric and apothecary equivalents for, 32*t*
 metric units of, 30, 30*f*
Wellbutrin, dosage calculation for, two-factor, 188, 188*f*

X

Xanax (alprazolam), dosage calculation for, 73, 73*f*
 one-factor, 167, 167*f*, 177, 177*f*

Y

Yield, 108

Z

Zantac
 administration of, as liquid, 79, 79*f*
 dosage calculation for, two-factor, 189, 189*f*
 intermittent infusion of, 123, 124
Zaroxolyn, dosage calculation for, 89, 89*f*
Zinacef, dosage calculation for, two-factor, 189, 189*f*
Zofran, dosage calculation for, two-factor, 187, 187*f*
Zovirax, dosage calculation for, two-factor, 188, 188*f*